MANAGEMENT OF HEALTH
AND FITNESS PROGRAMS

MANAGEMENT OF HEALTH AND FITNESS PROGRAMS

By

JAMES V. SULLIVAN, ED.D

Formerly Administrator of University of Southern Maine's
Health and Fitness Program—Lifeline
Director of Employee Health and Recreation Program
Professor of Health, Physical Education and Recreation
University of Southern Maine
Portland, Maine

With a Foreword by

Richard J. Clarey, PH.D.

Dean of School of Business,
Economics and Management
University of Southern Maine
Portland, Maine

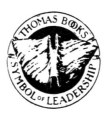

CHARLES C THOMAS • PUBLISHER
Springfield • Illinois • U.S.A.

Published and Distributed Throughout the World by

CHARLES C THOMAS • PUBLISHER
2600 South First Street
Springfield, Illinois 62794-9265

© *1990 by* CHARLES C THOMAS • PUBLISHER

ISBN 0-398-05651-X

Library of Congress Catalog Card Number: 89-37055

With THOMAS BOOKS *careful attention is given to all details of manufacturing
and design. It is the Publisher's desire to present books that are satisfactory as to their
physical qualities and artistic possibilities and appropriate for their particular use.*
THOMAS BOOKS *will be true to those laws of quality that assure a good name
and good will.*

Printed in the United States of America
SC-R-3

Library of Congress Cataloging-in-Publication Data

Sullivan, James V. (James Vincent)
    Management of health and fitness programs / by James V. Sullivan ;
with a foreword by Richard J. Clarey.
        p.   cm.
    Includes bibliographical references (p.   ).
    ISBN 0-398-05651-X
    1. Physical education and training—Administration. 2. Physical
fitness. 3. Occupational health services—Management. 4. Working
class—Physical training.   I. Title.
GV343.5.S85   1990
613.7′1—dc20   89-37055
                                                                              CIP

*This book is dedicated
to my wife, Ruth . . .
for without her it never
would have been written.*

FOREWORD

America's love affair with health and fitness, which blossomed in the seventies, continues unabated as the decade of the nineties arrives. Activities which were viewed 20 years ago as fads engaged in by a few stalwart ex-athletes or sporadic attempts by middle-aged sun worshippers to fit into last year's swimsuits have become part of the everyday life for millions of us. American Sports Data reports that there are more than 12 million runners in the U.S. alone. The Association for Fitness in Business has over 2,000 organization members who sponsor corporate fitness programs. Just 10 years ago, the membership numbered 25.

While a thorough analysis of the causes of this growing concern for our health and fitness is beyond the objectives or the expertise of this writer, certainly the aging of the population, a better educated and informed public, and the increased focus of the medical community on preventive medicine have played key roles in making us more aware of the dangers to our health posed by a sedentary or stressful life-style. Today, we need to be responsible for our own state of health and to take the steps necessary to avoid the diseases of inactivity.

Corporations and other organizations share this concern for health and fitness with each of us, for slightly different reasons. Rising costs of health insurance and workers' compensation insurance, reduced productivity due to absenteeism, an aging work force, and the spectre of all those Japanese workers exercising every morning are thoughts which do not make it any easier for a manager in a global economy to get a good night's rest. Furthermore, several U.S. assessment centers have conducted research on managers and found that effective managers are more likely to be able to sustain a high energy level throughout the day than their less effective counterparts.

The evidence which suggests the strategic importance of health and fitness-related activities to individual and organizational well-being is simply too overwhelming to ignore. That's why this book is so timely and so necessary. Individuals and organizations need to manage their health and fitness with the same effectiveness and efficiency that they bring to the management of other affairs, perhaps even more so.

There are few people more qualified on the subject of the management of health and fitness programs than James Sullivan. "Doc," as he is known, was responsible for designing and managing what has become the largest comprehensive health and fitness program in Maine and which has served as a model for many others throughout the country. Reaching thousands each year, the program has spread to private industry and other organizations and contains components for people of all ages and all degrees of fitness.

In this book, Doc Sullivan has brought together the concepts, the practices, and the principles vital to sound management in any undertaking and applied them to health and fitness programs. The result is a basic primer for managers in any organization contemplating a health and fitness program and for individuals considering a career in this important and rapidly growing field.

RICHARD J. CLAREY

PREFACE

Since the role of management is becoming increasingly significant in determining the success of health and fitness programs, the manner in which these programs are organized, structured, and supervised determines whether or not planned goals and objectives are met. Although management per se is now considered a science, health and fitness program management is relatively new. But regardless of where health and fitness programs are located, management plays a major role if these programs are to succeed.

The idea for writing this book stems from my fifteen years' experience in health and fitness program management and encouragement from the Dean of the School of Business, Economics and Management at the University of Southern Maine.

This book is organized into five parts. Part I, "Learning About Health and Fitness Program Management," has an introduction to program management and to the health and fitness manager. Part II, "Planning the Health and Fitness Program," familiarizes the reader with the manager's role; planning, design and content of the program; and suggested policies. Part III, "Organizing the Health and Fitness Program," provides information on the staff, facilities, and equipment for the health and fitness program. Part IV, "Leading the Health and Fitness Program," examines human resources, financial considerations and marketing, and medical and legal considerations. Part V, "Controlling the Health and Fitness Program," deals with evaluating the program and the future of health and fitness programs.

Acknowledgments

No book is exclusively the product of the individual whose name appears on its title page, since the author is influenced by other persons with whom he or she comes in contact.

The University of Southern Maine's School of Business, Economics and Management provided me with an ideal setting for the writing of this book. I would like to recognize the contributions of Dean Richard Clarey, Dr. John Voyer, Dr. Richard Grover, and Dr. Charles Greene.

Other persons at the University of Southern Maine helped me with specific topics on which they are experts: Dr. Robert Goettel, Paul Rogers, Larry Braziel, George Hackett, Bob Folsom, Len Jordan, Peter Allen, Ellen van Haasteren, the library staff, and Richard Emerson, an attorney in the city of Portland.

A special thanks is extended to Jenny Reed, Pam Baker, and Don Presnell.

James V. Sullivan

CONTENTS

PART IV.

Leading the Health and
Fitness Program

PART V.

Controlling the Health and
Fitness Program

MANAGEMENT OF HEALTH AND FITNESS PROGRAMS

PART I
LEARNING ABOUT HEALTH AND
FITNESS PROGRAM MANAGEMENT

Chapter I

INTRODUCTION TO HEALTH
AND FITNESS PROGRAM MANAGEMENT

PHILOSOPHY OF HEALTH AND FITNESS

Philosophy is concerned with the process of pursuing the beliefs, values and truths in ourselves. It recognizes the interrelationship between people and their environment and attempts to unify these two into an efficient and harmonious whole.

When people look at themselves as philosophers, they seek answers to basic questions as: Why am I living? Am I as healthy as I could be? Am I as physically fit as I could be? How can I improve my health and fitness level?

Personnel associated with the health profession have a philosophy which emphasizes the belief that any person can improve his or her health, if motivated to do so, by following, on a regular basis, the common practices that lead to good health. In addition, fitness professionals have a philosophy which stresses the truth that any person, regardless of age, sex or physical condition can reach an acceptable level of physical fitness if he or she makes a commitment to do so. The key words in these philosophies are *motivation* and *commitment.*

The words "health" and "fitness" can be defined in different ways. The most widely accepted definition of *health* in contemporary times comes from the World Health Organization, which defines health as "a state of complete physical, mental and social well-being and not merely the absence of disease or infirmity."[1] Obviously, a person's mental processes are an important influence on the way the individual acts, both physically and socially.

Basically, there are five types of fitness: emotional, mental, physical, social, and spiritual. But fitness as used in this book refers to physical only. Thus, *fitness* is defined as a quality, state of being, or condition that

---

1. World Health Organization, *The First Ten Years of the World Health Organization* (Geneva: World Health Organization, 1958), p. 459.

5

people possess or can develop when the body, mind, and spirit are all in proper balance and in harmony.

Upon close examination of the definitions for health and fitness, one can readily discover that they are quite similar. And, as a matter of fact, some authorities use these words interchangeably because, as people get involved in health programs, they invariably seek to improve their physical condition as well, and vice versa. For example, an individual may enroll in a smoking-cessation program and start jogging, or start jogging and enroll in a smoking-cessation program.

Meaning, Importance and Sources
of Philosophy of Health and Fitness

In recent years, there has been a dramatic increase in people's awareness of the intrinsic values of health and fitness. Yet, many people do not understand what health and fitness really mean because the words have different meanings to different people. Although a philosophy of health and fitness can be clearly stated, it has no real meaning or purpose unless people realize the benefits derived from being healthy and physically fit. For some people, *health* connotes freedom from headaches and fatigue. For others, health implies freedom from illness and disease. And for still others, health means faithfully adhering to all the common health guidelines.

For some, *fitness* means participating in a sport or recreational activity such as tennis or racquetball; for others, it denotes simply participating in some type of structured physical fitness program. And, for still others, fitness means walking, jogging, or weight training a few times a week.

In order for individuals to begin to see the importance of philosophies which relate to health and fitness, they need only to be aware of the diseases and problems which confront the population. These diseases are common: coronary heart disease, hypertension, obesity, diabetes, functional postural difficulties, chronic obstructive lung disease, migraines, insomnia, ulcers and psychological disorders. Research has shown that practicing good health habits and exercising regularly may alleviate some of these diseases and problems.

Talking and writing about the importance of the philosophies of health and fitness is one thing, but convincing and motivating people that there are benefits to be gained by practicing these philosophies can be a difficult task. Some may never be convinced that being in good health and being physically fit are important and may extend their life spans, while others will readily accept these philosophies and put them into action. After all, good health is something that cannot be bought; each of us is responsible for his or her own state of health.

Basically, there are three major sources from which a philosophy may originate: a personal philosophy of life, a philosophy of health, and a philosophy of fitness.

It would be impossible to have a philosophy of health and fitness disassociated from a person's philosophy of life. The beliefs, ideals, and values that individuals possess, their attitudes, feelings, and reactions to people give them direction to their lives. Lifelong objectives may be developed which can be used as guides for changing life-styles.

A personal philosophy of life may be difficult to express in writing; however, this assignment is recommended. It does, however, clarify that which a person actually thinks, believes, and lives. People may be surprised to discover that what they are presently doing and what their life objectives are, if written down and analyzed, can actually be used as guidelines for shaping their personal philosophies of life. It is much more beneficial for individuals to evaluate and modify their personal philosophy of life than have another person perform this task for them.

People should develop sound philosophies of health and of fitness to serve as directional guides and commitments to carry out these philosophies. A person's philosophy of health and fitness is usually the result of his or her experiences. For example, if a person has never experienced how much better one feels after losing a good amount of extra weight or has never experienced an aquatic fitness program, he or she has no basis for establishing a philosophy of health and of fitness. Although experiences will vary, they are the foundation upon which people can formulate their philosophies.

After individuals have formulated their health and fitness philosophies, they should evaluate their present life-styles; for the way people live has a profound effect on their mental and physical health. As mentioned previously, a sound philosophy that is expressed only in theory is worthless unless it is practiced continuously throughout a person's life span.

The philosophy of fitness is interrelated with the philosophy of health. Actually, being physically fit is often considered synonymous with being healthy. Perhaps of paramount importance is the fact that people must be educated as to the what's, how's, and when's of health and fitness.

Admittedly, many people lack both the philosophy and incentive to practice good health habits and to become involved in physical activity. Some people know what constitutes good health but tend to ignore their health for unknown reasons. And others shy away from any type of physical activity for reasons such as "I'm too lazy," "I'm in good enough physical shape already," "I don't have the time," or "I don't know how to exercise."

Without a sound philosophy of health and of fitness, a person has no course to follow to attain good health and physical well-being. There are within all human beings inward and outward drives which may be weak or strong, good or bad. These drives may not correlate with the objectives. Thus, the drives may be strong, but the objectives weak, or vice versa. Therefore, a sound philosophy of health and of fitness requires both drives and objectives.

WHAT IS MANAGEMENT?

One would be hard pressed not to find the definition of the word "management"* in any textbook on this subject. Writers and authorities in the field of management have given various definitions to the word; however, they all focus on the nature and importance of the management process. Perhaps the most often used meaning of the word is getting work accomplished through other persons.

Longnecker and Pringle put forth their definition of management that seems appropriate for use in this book:

> Management is the process of acquiring and combining human, financial, and physical resources to attain the organization's primary goal of producing a product or service desired by some segment of society. This process is essential to the functioning of all organizations— profit and nonprofit; essential resources must be acquired and combined in some way to produce an output.[2]

Although management may go unnoticed in many cases, it is an integral part of all organizations. Moreover, an organization, whether small or large, could not function without some type of management. Furthermore, management reaches into all phases of an organization

---

*In common usage, the term "management" is synonymous with "administration."

2. Justin G. Longnecker and Charles D. Pringle, *Management*, 5th ed. (Columbus, OH: Charles E. Merrill Co., 1981), p. 5.

and is essential if coordination is to be achieved as people work together either to produce a product or perform a service.

THE PROCESS AND ESSENTIAL SKILLS OF MANAGEMENT

A comprehensive review of literature related to management reveals that authorities in the field disagree on the number of, and interpretation of, the elements involved in the management process. However, for the purposes of this book, it seems best to identify and briefly define five basic management functions:

Planning: The management function concerned with defining goals for future organizational performance and deciding on the tasks and resource use needed to attain them. *Goals* typically fall into nine categories: profitability, physical and financial resources, productivity, marketing, innovation, management development, worker attitudes and performance, social responsibility, and stockholder responsibility. Planning is a conscious, purposeful, analytical process carried out in advance of action. It is often done by skilled, specialized staff. The emphasis is usually on the *integration* of organizational activities. Plans are often highly articulated in formal documents.

Organizing: The management function concerned with assigning tasks, grouping tasks into departments, and allocating resources to departments. Organizations may be *functionally* organized, where departments are founded on the skills of their members. They may also be *divisionally* organized, where a large organization is broken down into smaller, self-contained units clustered around customer or client needs. Organizing also includes coordinating the members of the organization. This includes vertical coordination, using levels of hierarchy, for example, and *horizontal* coordination, using liaison devices like task forces.

Leading: The management function that involves the use of influence to motivate employees to achieve the organization's goals. Managers are responsible for making high-quality decisions, and for making sure that those decisions are acceptable to the organization's employees. Leaders use intrinsic and extrinsic methods to *motivate* employees to fulfill organizational goals. In most medium and large organizations, leadership also means using *power* and *influence* in an enlightened way to gain employees' acceptance of methods designed to achieve goals.

Controlling: The management function concerned with monitoring employees' activities, keeping the organization on track toward its

Note: "Organizations," as used in this book, refers to businesses, industries, hospitals, colleges, universities, governmental agencies, health clubs, fitness clubs, YMCA's, YWCA's, and other similar profit-making and not-for-profit organizations.

goals, and making corrections as needed. The first step in this process is the establishment of *performance standards*. The next step is the *measurement* and *monitoring* of actual performance. This function typically involves the design and implementation of *systems* for monitoring performance. The final step in the control cycle is *feedback* to correct performance. There are three types of control. *Market* control uses price-cost comparisons to evaluate performance, and it requires price competition so that price reflects the true value of outputs. *Bureaucratic* control (the most common) is the use of rules, regulations, policies, hierarchy, documentation, and other mechanisms to standardize behavior. *Clan* control is the use of values, commitment, traditions, trust, and shared beliefs to control behavior.

Staffing: The management function concerned with obtaining, developing, evaluating, compensating and retaining human resources for the organization. This function typically begins with *human resource planning* to ascertain present and future needs for employees. The process continues with *recruitment and selection* of the needed staff. New employees must be inducted into the organization using *orientation*. *Training* programs impart needed skills, while *development* programs prepare employees for broader responsibilities. *Compensation and benefits* must be managed as part of this basic function, and a vital part of any manager's job is *performance evaluation* of his or her employees. Lastly, managers must deal with *transfers* and *terminations*.[3]

Mondy, Holmes and Flippo have indicated that there are essential skills of management necessary at various levels—top, middle, and lower (supervisory)—in any organization. They identify and define these skills as follows:

Technical skill is "the ability to use specific knowledge, methods, or techniques in performing work. . . . "

Communication skill is "the ability to provide information orally and in written form to others in the organization for the purpose of achieving desired results. . . . "

Human skill is "the ability of a manager to understand, work with, and get along with other people. . . . "

Analytical skill is "the ability of the manager to use logical and scientific approaches or techniques in the analyses of problems and business opportunities. . . . "

Decision-making skill is "the manager's skill in selecting a course of action from several alternatives. . . . "

---

3. Personal communication with Dr. John Voyer, Assistant Professor of Business Administration, University of Southern Maine, Portland, Maine, October, 1987.

Conceptual skill is "the ability of the manager to understand the complexities of the overall organization and how each department contributes to the accomplishment of the firm's objectives. . . ."[4]

Democratic-Participative Management

A style of management that permits and encourages its employees, whether individuals or groups, to offer their ideas, opinions, and thinking on appropriate matters or problems which affect the organization preceding the decision-making process is called democratic-participative management.

Without exception, managers of these organizations are deeply concerned with employee productivity and job satisfaction. Accordingly, the following are values related to democratic-participative management:

- Increased acceptability of management's ideas
- Increased cooperation with members of management and staff
- Reduced turnover
- Reduced absenteeism
- Reduced complaints and grievances
- Greater acceptance of changes
- Improved attitudes toward the job and the organization[5]

Although there are values related to democratic-participative management, there are some limitations. When organizations permit their employees to participate in the decision-making process, the requirements they must meet include "(1) sufficient time; (2) adequate ability and interest on the part of the participants; and (3) restrictions generated by the present structure and system."[6]

THE NEED FOR HEALTH AND FITNESS PROGRAM MANAGEMENT

The need for management is imperative as soon as the organization makes the decision to implement a health and fitness program. Management becomes necessary if both the organization and the program goals and objectives are to be realized. When organizations are

---

4. R. Wayne Mondy, Robert E. Holmes. and Edwin R. Flippo, *Management: Concepts and Practices*, 2nd. ed. (Boston, MA: Allyn and Bacon, Inc.. 1983), pp. 14–16.

5. Ibid., p. 421.

6. Ibid., p. 422.

ready to start a program, usually the first person to be hired is the manager.* Although this person will assume all the managerial responsibilities, he or she may also be involved with other duties dependent upon the type(s) and number(s) of programs that will be offered.

Once a health or fitness program is completed and has been a success, the manager may either repeat it or start a new one. Obviously, as a comprehensive health and fitness program expands, so then will managerial responsibilities increase. As a result, a manager's duties may become too time-consuming. If the manager becomes overburdened with work, the time has come to hire either a full-time or a part-time staff** member. Regardless of which of these staff members is employed, the coordinating responsibilities necessitate management. Simply stated, someone needs to be in charge to take the leadership role, and that person is the manager.

Any organization that decides to start a health and fitness program expects to see dramatic growth over a period of time. But the only way this can be assured is to have the management of the program in "the right hands" from the very beginning, as the need for sound management is essential.

HEALTH AND FITNESS PROGRAM MANAGEMENT

When the terms "health," "fitness," and "program management," as used in this book, are combined, they refer to a process whereby managers working with other professionals assist individuals in attaining good health and optimum levels of physical fitness. This process encourages changes in life-style by providing health and fitness instruction, health and fitness counseling, facilities, and equipment so that individuals are given an opportunity to participate in various health and fitness programs or components.†

Health and fitness components do not automatically operate efficiently and effectively. Their success depends heavily upon the type of leader-

---

Note: If the organization has a union(s), its (their) representative(s) should work closely with the health and fitness manager.

*The word "manager" as used in this book is synonymous with "director."

**"Staff," as used here, consists of all instructional personnel who work for the health and fitness manager.

†The words "programs" or "components" are used interchangeably as part of a comprehensive health and fitness program.

ship known as management. When health and fitness management is effective, so then will be the program. It follows that health and fitness program management actually means molding and guiding human behavior toward achieving desired goals and objectives.

The importance of health and fitness program management cannot be overemphasized. These programs can determine, to a large extent, the quality of life for a given population; and their managers, as a class, determine this quality.

Admittedly, health and fitness programs can fail because of inadequate funds, facilities, equipment, and staff and for many other reasons. They often fail, however, because the basic management functions are performed poorly or not at all. Sound management can make the difference between a successful or unsuccessful health and fitness program.

SUMMARY

People who live by the philosophy of optimum health and fitness have a positive outlook on life, since they realize that not only the span of life but also the quality of life depend upon their mental and physical well-being.

If a person were to look up the words "health" and "fitness," he or she would discover that the definitions are quite similar; and in contemporary times, the terms health and fitness are often used interchangeably. However, knowing the meanings of the words is one thing, but putting their meanings into practice is another.

The three major sources from which a philosophy originates—a personal philosophy of life, a philosophy of health, and a philosophy of fitness—can give a person direction in life. Having a philosophy of life is valueless unless it is put into action.

Although management can be defined in several ways, the meanings are all centered on the management process. Because management is contiguous on all parts of an organization, as people come together the coordination of their efforts is imperative.

The process of management includes planning, organizing, staffing, leading, and controlling. Clearly, if managers do not possess sufficient skills, they are bound to be unsuccessful.

Democratic-participative management allows employees to offer their suggestions, opinions, and ideas. There are several related values, but there are some limitations to this type of management style.

No one can dispute the need for good health and fitness program management. Good program management requires that the person in charge possess both knowledge and skills. If the program is to grow, then its management must be strong and effective.

The key to success to any health and fitness program is effective management. The management process, as used within the context of a health and fitness program, is essential to the functioning of the program itself. Without sound management, the program will not survive.

Chapter II

THE HEALTH AND FITNESS MANAGER

CHOOSING THE MANAGER

Once an organization has made the decision to offer a health and fitness program, the choosing of a manager must follow. Although the interviewing process can consume a great amount of time, the choosing of the person best qualified for the position is certainly worth the effort. When the manager is chosen judiciously, he or she should start the program on the right course. The leader will also set a certain type of leadership style.

What Are the Leadership Styles?

It seems prudent then, in this chapter, to begin with a thorough discussion of the various types of leadership styles. As a resultant of this section will come a recommendation as to the style most appropriate for health and fitness managers. Therefore, the following information may prove helpful:

Managers may be categorized by the way in which they view their authority and how they use it. Managers must first and foremost be recognized as leaders and be accepted by their subordinates.

The type of leadership style employed by the manager has been the subject of much study, research, and theory. Actually, there are several leadership style theories, but perhaps the most widely known is the Managerial Grid® developed by Blake and Mouton.[7] Their Grid is illustrated in a chart that appears below.

The two key dimensions found in the Blake and Mouton Managerial Grid that influence all managers are "concern for people" and "concern for production." Thus, managers can be labeled according to the degree to which they are concerned with people, with production, or both.

---

7. Robert R. Blake and Jane Srygley Mouton, *The Managerial Grid, III.* 3rd ed. (Houston, TX: Gulf Publishing Co., 1985), p. 12. Reproduced by permission.

Figure 1

Managerial Grid

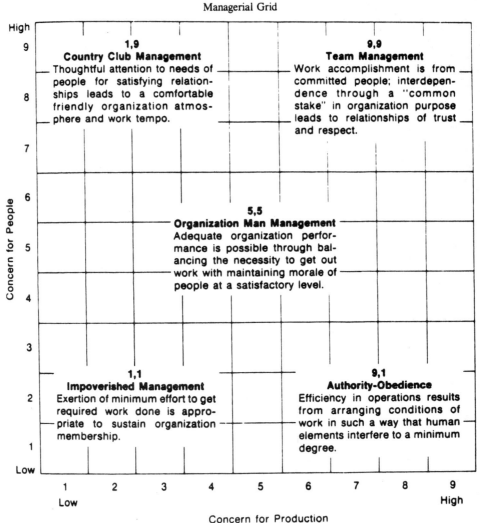

On the *horizontal axis,* concern for production, leaders are started on a 1- to 9-point scale; 1 represents the lowest score and 9 the highest. On the *vertical axis,* concern for people, leaders are also scored on a 1- to 9-point scale; 1 represents the lowest and 9 the highest. To avoid any confusion, it should be noted that the first digit stands for concern for production, the second digit for concern for people. For example, a location on the chart of 9,1 would rank the manager high in concern for production but low in concern for people. At the other end of the scale, a location of 1,9 would rank the manager low in concern for production but high in his or her concern for people. As one can readily see, predicated on the grid, managers who score high in concern for both production and people are classified as 9,9; thus, they are the most effective leaders. Furthermore, because health and fitness managers are people- and service-oriented, it is recommended that they all strive to become classified as 9,9's. (In this case, service is substituted for production.) Ideally, all managers should work toward and develop a 9,9 orientation.

In the grid, there are 81 possible combinations for the two key dimensions, concern for people and concern for production; however, Blake and Mouton identify only the five major leadership styles as follows:

- 1,1. *Impoverished Management* —The manager de-emphasizes concerns for both people and production.
- 9,1. *Authority-Obedience* —The manager concentrates on production and has little concern for people.
- 1,9. *Country Club Management* —The manager is concerned with people and has minimal concern for production.
- 5,5. *Organization Man Management* —The manager attempts to balance work output with satisfactory people relations.
- 9,9. *Team Management* —The manager has high concern for both production and people.

Any discussion of leadership styles would be incomplete without mentioning the results of recent studies with reference to managers' physical condition. It has been clearly pointed out above that not only do all managers need to strive to be team managers but also to become physically fit in order to possess high energy levels and work effectiveness. Additionally, managers who are in good physical condition are less likely to be absent from work.

Where Do Health and Fitness Managers Come From?

Because of the rapid growth of health and fitness programs, the position of managers has evolved over a relatively short period of time. Regardless of the newness of both programs and managerial positions, the fact remains that the manager's background and qualifications must coincide with the organization's present and future program offerings. After all, the program dictates the types of backgrounds and qualifications managers need. Yet, as with other managerial positions, there are no universally accepted standards and certification requirements for health and fitness managerial positions. Some organizations offer only health education programs, while others offer only fitness programs; and some offer only physical recreation. However, it is recommended that organizations offer both health and fitness programs whenever possible.

Health and fitness managers are usually graduates of colleges and universities that grant degrees under a variety of titles: health studies, health education, health science, public health, health administration, nutrition, health/fitness, exercise physiology, exercise science, and exercise science/health maintenance. Also, a degree in health, physical education, and recreation, with a concentration in fitness, is also quite common. Regardless of the degree designation, a series of business management courses must become an integral part of the academic program.

It is imperative that prospective managers have scientific and technical training in both health and fitness and in managerial training. With respect to the scientific and technical training in the area of health and fitness, the following courses can prove helpful: human anatomy and physiology, personal health, community health, environmental health, mental health, health counseling, public health administration, nutrition/weight management, substance abuse, exercise physiology, kinesiology, biomechanics, motor learning, sports medicine, fitness counseling, muscular relaxation, first aid safety, and fitness evaluation and assessment. The business management courses that can prove helpful are financial and managerial accounting, principles of economics, business finance, principles of management, and marketing. Additionally, courses in human relations and communications have been proven to be beneficial. Advanced degree graduate programs can offer prospective managers further specialization, which often leads to certification and enhanced career opportunities.

In addition to professional preparation in health and fitness, managers in these positions can gain a body of knowledge by attending institutes, conferences, seminars and workshops. Moreover, the availability of literature and books on health and fitness is increasing rapidly. Furthermore, if an organization is conducting only fitness programs, some managers who are interested may wish to review the test given by the American College of Sports Medicine.

If interested in pursuing a career in health and fitness program management, one should review health and fitness programs conducted in various organizations and, particularly, the training and qualifications necessary for becoming a manager. It will come as no surprise that the majority of managers will have earned any one of the degrees previously mentioned in this section. If not, they have taken relevant course work in the areas of health, nutrition, physical education, exercise science, and business management.

What Do Health and Fitness Managers Do?

Nowhere in the literature will one find total consistency as to what health and fitness managers actually do. The responsibility of managers varies from one organization to another, depending upon the goals and objectives of the organization, the size of the organization itself, the number of different health and fitness components presently offered and planned for the future, the number of qualified staff, and the availability of both indoor and outdoor facilities.

The duties of a health and fitness manager that are recognized in most organizations are listed below. He or she

- Is an innovator
- Acts as a role model
- Builds a harmonious working environment
- Communicates both orally and in writing with the staff
- Is skillful in interpersonal relationships
- Makes all necessary decisions
- Establishes short- and long-range plans with help from the staff
- Administers a health and fitness program pertaining to risk factor modification and intervention
- Assists in the development of program content of all health and fitness classes in accordance with program policies, rules, and procedures and continuously updates program contents according to the latest developments in the field of health education and exercise science
- Markets the program effectively
- Coordinates all health and fitness programs and activities
- Schedules and monitors the actual health and fitness instructional hours
- Is responsible for the formulation of all program policies and sees that they are carried out

- Assists in the development and management of in-service training in health and fitness for all instructional personnel
- Recruits staff as needed
- Hires health instructors and fitness instructors
- Hires resource personnel and/or consultants, if necessary
- Works closely with union leader(s), if present, on all health and fitness programs
- Supervises all health instructors and fitness instructors
- Is competent in evaluation and research
- Provides a system for ongoing evaluation of all health and fitness staff and programs
- Assists in establishing emergency medical policies
- Assists in establishing safety precautions for all instructional programs
- Is responsible for all legal aspects of the health and fitness program
- Develops a budget and implements and controls it, once it is approved
- Oversees the usage of computers, if available
- Supervises office personnel
- Requests purchases of health and fitness supplies and equipment
- Is responsible for the cleanliness and maintenance of the facilities, if they are on-site, and
- Expands the program, when feasible.

In order to better understand what health and fitness managers do, the day-to-day responsibilities of Jane Day and James Day are discussed below. It is important to remember, however, that each individual may never repeat the same work on any other day.

Jane Day's organization employs 150 people and has approximately 70 participants. She has one part-time staff who instructs health education classes (Jane's background is in exercise science). Jane, on a day-to-day basis, does the following: answers mail and memoranda, writes letters and memoranda, makes phone calls, teaches two fitness classes, does individual fitness testing and screening, meets with her immediate supervisor, meets with her instructor to plan a new program, and develops a budget for the proposed program.

By contrast, James Day's organization employs 500 people and has approximately 265 participants. (James' background is in public health.) He employs one full-time and two part-time staff who teach two health education classes and four fitness classes. They also do all the fitness testing and screening. James Day's work consists of answering mail and memoranda, writing letters and memoranda, answering phone calls, making phone calls, meeting with his immediate supervisor, meeting with his staff to coordinate and schedule classes, meeting with his staff to plan new programs, supervising the staff and the secretary, using the computer, preparing all requisitions to purchase supplies, developing a budget for the proposed program, checking the budget, and checking the equipment and facility.

Where are Health and Fitness Managers Going?

At this point in time, it is impossible to predict the future of health and fitness managers, because health and fitness programs are relatively new but increasing rapidly. Today, there have been no studies that focused specifically upon health and fitness managerial positions and the outlook for these types of jobs. As a result, there are no data available from which to draw conclusions as to where managers of health and fitness programs are going. What can be documented, however, is the number of organizations that have some type of fitness program. (Health education programs were not mentioned in the study, nor the number of corporations who employ full-time physical fitness directors.)

The literature has also pointed out the small percentage of major corporations that have fitness programs and predicted that by 1990 there will be a significant increase in these types of programs in organizations. But it is interesting to note that these so-called fitness programs were quite diversified. After all is said and done, health and fitness programs must have leaders and these are the managers. In other words, it is the increase of health and fitness programs and the expanding career opportunities for managers that will give some indication as to where health and fitness managers are going. Moreover, demographics indicate that in the future there will be more older people in our society who are concerned with their health and physical well-being.

In addition to the above considerations concerning the future of health and fitness managers, there are several other factors. Some of the following questions need to be answered before any accurate account can be made regarding the future of health and fitness managers:

- What is the future of the organization?
- What is the outlook for changes within the organization?

- How will a changing society, and a changing world of technology, affect the organization and, in turn, affect the program?
- What does the organization expect to gain from a health and fitness program?
- What are the ways a health and fitness program can help both the participant and the organization?
- What are the strategies to use to keep up the support from top management and the union(s), if present.

Perhaps the best approach to end this section is to say that health and fitness programs, as well as the managerial positions, are in a developmental stage, with many miles of road ahead. The success of any health and fitness program depends heavily upon the dedication and motivation of its manager, the continued strong support of the organization, and the union(s), if present.

SUMMARY

The choosing of a qualified manager is very important to an organization, since all managers should strive to be good leaders because they are the key individuals who can either make or break a health and fitness program. The Managerial Grid is widely recognized as a scale to rank managers according to their concern for both production and people. According to the developers of this grid, team management, which all managers should strive to attain, is the best leadership style.

Health and fitness program managers are usually graduates of colleges and universities that grant degrees in either the health or exercise science field. Organizations that are looking for a program manager should attempt to match the manager's background and qualifications to the present and future program(s) to be offered. There is a body of knowledge, both scientific and technical, that managers must acquire; but just as important is knowledge in the management field. Above and beyond professional preparation, managers can learn about the health and fitness field by attending conferences, seminars, and workshops on these subjects.

The duties of health and fitness managers vary from organization to organization, and there are no set standards as to managers' responsibilities. As a result, health and fitness managerial positions cannot be standardized within a specific job description. What does exist, however, is a list of managers' duties that are recognized by most organizations.

Because health and fitness programs are relatively new, studies that have been made indicate that both the organization and the participant will benefit. That being the case, managers are needed to provide leadership. However, there are several factors that affect the future of managerial positions, and questions need to be answered before any accurate prediction can be made regarding the future of health and fitness managers. Moreover, because of the changes that can occur in an organization, in society, and in the technological world, the future of program managers cannot be guaranteed.

PART II
PLANNING THE HEALTH AND
FITNESS PROGRAM

Chapter III

PLANNING THE HEALTH AND FITNESS PROGRAM: THE MANAGER'S ROLE

WHAT IS PLANNING?

Planning is a continuous process whereby a course of action for the future is established in which program goals and objectives are formulated and resources identified for achieving them. It is a required mental and intellectual function of management which should precede actual implementation. Moreover, any type of effective planning should include concepts, creative thinking, knowledge, and sound reasoning. Furthermore, by planning, decision making is molded into a framework which can lessen the choices which have come into focus. Thus, the manager's role in all planning efforts is of extreme importance.

Why Plan for Health and Fitness?

Without question, people are the most important resource of any organization. Although there have been dramatic growth and advancement in the field of technology, human resources must still be considered as the number one priority. In light of this truism, organizations more than ever before are beginning to promote the health and physical well-being of people.

The success of any health and fitness program depends heavily on good planning. Although it may be costly and time consuming, planning is an essential part of management. Poor planning, or lack of planning, is on a continuum from unsatisfactory performance to complete failure.

Insufficient personnel and/or lack of facilities, supplies and equipment can all be attributed to lack of planning. By careful and sensible planning, managers can avoid hasty actions and hurried decisions. Many managers have said that they do not have the time to spend on planning

27

because they are too busy doing more important tasks. This kind of thinking is not acceptable. For example, a carpenter could not, or would not, build a house without a blueprint to follow.

Much planning needs to be done in health and fitness programming if implementation is to go smoothly and effectively. Planning will provide direction and a sense of purpose. It minimizes risks, facilitates control, and prevents quick decisions. Thus, sound planning is the nucleus of good management.

Who Plans?

All health and fitness managers plan in one way or another. There are four common approaches; any one, or a combination thereof, may be utilized with respect to the number of individuals or committees involved in the planning process. However, regardless of the approach used, ultimately it is the sole responsibility of the manager to see that sound planning takes place. Thus, the following four different approaches to planning are explained:

• All planning is done solely by the manager. Although this method is time-consuming, it provides for complete control, inflexibility, and alleviation of conflict concerning change. Furthermore, this approach helps in the development of effective managers.

• Ideas and suggestions are solicited from instructors but are screened and finalized by the manager. This approach is popular because often "several minds are better than one"; yet complete control is retained by the manager.

• Instructors do all the planning but submit the plans to the manager for either rejection, approval, or modification. This approach relieves the manager of most of the planning effort and helps staff members gain knowledge in planning. The disadvantage, however, is that the plan will lack the manager's contributions and, consequently, may be viewed as unimportant.

• Committees or task forces can be formed and used for planning. These groups are composed of people from all parts and levels of an organization including union official(s), if present. In most cases, they generate sound ideas and suggestions because they take on the planning assignment as a personal obligation, an honor, and a task wherein they gain valuable experience. However, there is a possibility that they can spend a great deal of time discussing the information and still not formulate a tentative plan.[8]

When To Plan

The question of when to plan needs to be carefully considered in light of the meaning of planning, which was previously defined. Some confusion may arise between the meaning of planning and the answer to the question of the proper time to plan. The health and fitness manager and staff personnel involved should not put planning aside because they have a heavy work load. All programs require definite planning. For example, if a smoking-cessation program is to be implemented on a specific date, several months' planning is mandatory prior to its implementation.

Most health and fitness managers maintain that in order to formulate sound and effective plans, they must be free from any interruptions such as telephone calls and unscheduled visits from staff personnel. It is extremely difficult to think clearly and to concentrate on specific material when any type of interruption occurs.

Proper timing requires a definite beginning and a definite end to planning for any specific program, budget, or facility in order for the plan to be effective upon implementation. Having provided the answer as to when to plan, the manager must realize planning is always a continuous process, although it does not necessarily have to occur eight hours a day, five days a week, and twelve months a year.

Plans, however, can be differentiated according to arbitrary time spans: short, intermediate, and long-range plans. Short-range plans involve a time span of one year or less, intermediate-range plans cover a one- to five-year period, and long-range plans extend for five years or more.

Use of Staff in Planning

A good plan design begins with the selection of planning personnel, and it is the prudent health and fitness manager who utilizes his or her own staff, if available. Whether part-time or full-time, every member of a staff can be stimulated into usefulness if properly motivated. Stimulation and encouragement can produce valuable suggestions and ideas for

---

8. Adapted from George R. Terry and Stephen G. Franklin, *Principles of Management*, 8th ed. (Homewood. IL: Richard D. Irwin, Inc., 1982), pp. 174–175.

planning. The utilization of a staff in any planning efforts usually guarantees a plan that is well thought out. Furthermore, it gives staff members a feeling of "belonging" and of making a contribution to the program. By the same token, it will certainly limit or eliminate negative criticism and create an atmosphere of cooperation.

In small organizations that employ only a health and fitness manager and no staff, it is obvious that planning is solely his or her responsibility. However, the manager should seek help from volunteers within the organization or from the community. Of course, if funds are available, consultants can be hired to help work on various plans.

The questions that often arises are: What are the major characteristics of a good health and fitness planner? He or she is:

- Willing to learn
- Willing to work and be motivated
- Flexible
- Imaginative
- Creative
- Deep thinking
- Up-to-date on new developments
- Well read in the area of health and fitness promotion, and
- Committed to health and fitness promotion.

The following is an example of the use of personnel in planning and the best use of human resources within a health and fitness program: Jean J. is employed by an insurance company as a health and fitness instructor with a specialty in weight training. The manager has conducted a needs survey, and the results revealed that a weight training program is desired and that space is available within the building. Obviously, only weight training equipment needs to be purchased. Without question, Jean would be in on the planning of the proposed weight training component, since her expertise and experience will be valuable to the planning process.

TYPES OF PLANS

Generally speaking, health and fitness managers are involved with two types of plans: single-use or one-time use, and standing-use. The first type, *single-use plans*, is created for one specific situation and is not likely to be repeated. A few examples of these single-use plans are developing a health and fitness needs assessment, purchasing and location of weight training equipment, and location of staff offices. *Standing-use plans* include the policies, procedures, and rules* which will be used again and again as guidelines for the program. Since standing-use plans tend to be of more value to programs in relatively stable situations, they are utilized by virtually all types of organizations. A few examples of standing-use plans as related to programs are an in-service training plan for instructors, maintenance plan for weight training equipment, and a safety plan for both the participants and the facility, if in-house.

STRATEGIES IN HEALTH AND FITNESS PROGRAM PLANNING

With reference to planning, the word "strategy" is becoming very popular in the field of management. Therefore, it may be advisable to define the word "strategy," a term derived from military usage which describes the deployment of military personnel and equipment to achieve a military objective. In management usage, strategy is used in long-range planning as the ways and means of acquiring and utilizing resources to achieve established goals and objectives. Thus, plans and strategy are quite similar.

Trewatha and Newport have the following to say about the advantages of strategy planning:

> Not all managers believe that strategy planning is useful or even possible. Some suggest that the future is too complex and difficult to anticipate. Of course, perfect accuracy in forecasting is impossible since the future holds many uncertainties. But, what is likely to happen to an organization that does not try to understand those basic marketplace phenomena that both lead and force change? More than likely it will be blighted with troubles affecting survival and growth. Changes in society, the future impact of current decisions, and the complexity of governmental regulations, and the increased pressures of competition can hinder survival unless managers make strategic decisions. Surely, strategy planning can assist management in anticipating unfavorable factors and changing environments in which organizations must survive and grow.[9]

Although the above quote is directed more to an organization than to a program, its meaning has direct application to a health and fitness

---

*For more information on policies, procedures, and rules, see Chapter V.

9. Robert L. Trewatha and M. Gene Newport, *Management,* 3rd ed. (Homewood, IL: Richard D. Irwin, Inc., 1982), p. 121.

program. If any health and fitness program is to gain quality, stability, and growth, the manager must become involved in strategic planning. Regardless of the organization's mission, the participants are the benefactors of the program and this program must survive. Furthermore, strategy planning can lead to achieving the program's goals and objectives.

TYPES OF STRATEGIES[10]

There are four basic types of grand strategies available to managers: stability, internal growth, external growth, and retrenchment:

• *Stability* continues the health and fitness program in its present course of action. Organizations that have health and fitness programs tend to use this strategy most frequently for four reasons: (1) When the program is already perceived to be running smoothly and efficiently, (2) There is no risk in this course of action, (3) If there are no problems associated with the program, it is easier and more comfortable as a course of action, (4) It allows the health and fitness manager to spend more time on other strategies. It should be clearly understood that the choice of a stability strategy does not mean that the program is at a "standstill" posture. Instead, it is a continuation of the existing program which emphasizes quality and personal relationships.

• *Internal growth* as used in this book refers to expanding the health and fitness program and facilities at the present location and will mean more funding for staff, facilities, equipment and supplies. There are six reasons as to why managers should adopt the growth strategy: (1) Increase profits, (2) Increase enrollments, (3) Facilities are no longer adequate due to increased enrollments, (4) Lack of space for new equipment, (5) Demand for new programs, and (6) More accessible locations.

But growth of the program should occur only through a pattern of expanded existing health and fitness components or through the addition of new components. In either case, growth is a more risky strategy to pursue than stability, and the pressure on the manager is greater.

Growth is necessary if the program is to continue for a long time; stability can mean the program will have a short-term success but long-term cessation. Many health and fitness managers equate growth with accomplishment. Organizations, the program, and their participants benefit from growth strategy. Many managers wish to be known as making a contribution to the organization so they are motivated to gamble and therefore choose a growth strategy. Of course risk is less with a stability strategy. When the program shows growth, it attracts

---

10. Voyer, personal communication.

more employees and can also be used as an added benefit for those who seek employment in a particular organization.

• *External growth* refers to the aspirations of some organizations to expand externally. This expansion may be accomplished in two different ways: they may conduct their programs at other sites in various locations or they may actually merge through acquisition of other organizations that have similar or related programs. Therefore, external growth becomes an important strategy.

• *Retrenchment* indicates that a decision is made to level-off, reduce enrollment, and strive to maintain and improve the quality of the program. This strategy is used less frequently and is least popular of all strategies. When this strategy is pursued, it is an admission that the program was not a success and should be viewed as a "last resort."

STEPS IN STRATEGIC HEALTH AND FITNESS PROGRAM PLANNING

The success of any health and fitness program depends heavily on how much time and effort are devoted to its planning. If the program is to grow, keeping in mind that a program is voluntary, there are specific steps that should be used in developing a sound strategy to follow. These steps are used as a basis of managerial planning.

The first step is to identify specific goals and objectives to be achieved. This step requires an analysis of the target audience so that an anticipated number of potential participants may be realized. Goals and objectives must be operationally defined so that they have a greater chance of attainment.

Second, a program must be developed that will focus upon its established goals and objectives. Emphasis is placed on (1) encouraging participants to modify their health habits, (2) creating change of participants' life-style through the program, and (3) avoiding attrition by motivating and encouraging participants to continue in the program.

The third step involves a program structure. Without question, program structure is of utmost importance if all components are to function smoothly and effectively; a must, if established goals and objectives are to be attained. The design of the structure should be such that managers have ample time for strategic program planning, which, in turn, may help them make faster decisions.

A fourth step requires employing staff personnel who possess the abilities and skills to make the program a success. In many situations, staff may be either full-time or part-time personnel. Competent personnel make a health and fitness program a success—not facilities, equipment, supplies, or even money.

The fifth step involves spending time on strategic matters rather than on day-to-day activities. Frequently, managers of health and fitness programs spend much of their time dealing with matters that should be delegated. Obviously, these managers are managing large programs in large organizations. The constant handling of these day-to-day situations results in not enough time available for strategic planning. Instead, they spend valuable time and energy engaging in daily crises. Of course, it is necessary for the managers to face emergencies. The key to this step is for managers to channel energies into what the program should be doing for the participants.

The final strategic step in planning is an evaluation of all the given strategies so that changes can be made where and when necessary. Without question, health and fitness programs will undergo changes. Therefore, the manager should be ready to confront these changes in a systematic fashion. Managers will find that their programs are more likely to be successful when strategies are developed systematically and changed when necessary.[11]

STRATEGIC ALTERNATIVES IN HEALTH AND FITNESS PROGRAM PLANNING

The following discussion provides managers with various strategic alternatives that may be utilized in health and fitness program planning. Managers should find comfort in the knowledge that there are strategic alternatives available. These alternatives may help managers to confront any unforeseen changes with a positive frame of mind that can result in continuing the program on a high-quality level and, by doing so, help the organization and its participants. Any strategic plan, to be successful, needs to be adjusted to the anticipated reactions of the staff. Plans will be difficult to implement if they do not take into consideration the reactions of those affected. Terry and Franklin in their book, *Principles of Management,* list ten strategic alternatives devised by Professor L.C. Sorrell of the University of Chicago which should be useful to the health and fitness manager in any planning effort. Regardless of the size of the organization, the following strategies can prove helpful:

---

11. Adapted from Trewatha and Newport, *Management,* pp. 125–126.

1. *Camel's head in the tent:* This implies that sometimes a small portion of a plan may be acceptable, whereas an entire plan may be unacceptable. In many instances a staff will agree that a part or parts of a particular plan can be offered and, in all probability, will be successful until the entire original plan is put into action.

2. *Sowing seed on fertile ground:* Obviously, to propose a finalized plan to a staff may meet with acceptance by some and rejection by others. On the other hand, a much better approach is to offer a tentative plan and discover who on the staff are the allies and who are the disinterested members. By utilizing this approach, those individuals who favor the plan are quickly identified. After the staff members who are in favor of the plan have been selected, they need to be indoctrinated as to the benefits and values of the plan, answering any questions they may have and thus creating more enthusiasm and momentum for its implementation. By selling the plan to those in favor, the plan is developed, and those disinterested staff members who have different viewpoints and opinions may be won over so that eventually a sufficient number of the staff will agree to accept the plan once it is presented in its final form.

3. *Mass concentrated offensive:* This strategy favors getting the total plan implemented at one time and as quickly as possible. In contrast to the gradual penetration strategy, the mass concentrated offensive calls for an all-out effort. The philosophy which underlies this approach stresses the need to put the initial plan into action, discard any irregularities, and carry on with those activities that have proven to be successful.

4. *Confuse the issue:* This technique calls for concentrated effort to be employed that distracts the attention of the staff by raising a series of questions which are unrelated to the major issues under consideration. This theory may be utilized when the staff's concentration should be focused on the acceptable issues and on downplaying the controversial issues.

5. *Use strong tactics only when necessary:* The key to this strategy is to use only as much pressure as absolutely necessary to reach the desired goal. Sufficiently strong tactics and power should be kept in reserve for any future emergencies. Sometimes an extra push is required, but it should be used only for special events or when the tentative plan is under consideration.

6. *Pass the buck:* This technique calls for transferring or placing the

responsibility on some other staff member. When a plan is finalized, it is possible to hand over the disliked tasks to others. This maneuver is accomplished in such a manner that the blame is placed on another person.

7. *Time is a great healer:* Oftentimes, some plans may have a better chance for success after the staff has had an opportunity to see the total plan in perspective. This is sometimes referred to as a "cooling-off" period. When difficulties arise, time has a way of helping the staff to find solutions. It has been said that "haste makes waste"; basically, this is the philosophy which this strategy is predicated upon. For some, it is a mistake to make hurried decisions. Putting off the action for a period of time may eliminate some of the problems. The key words to many planning strategies are "time" and "timing."

8. *Strike while the iron is hot:* Once a plan has been finalized and accepted, implement it as quickly as possible. Take full advantage when the situation is propitious. Quick action today can prevent opposition or difficulties tomorrow. To get a plan under way, immediate action is essential. Procrastination may be a spoiler.

9. *Two heads are better than one:* This technique stresses the importance of soliciting all the assistance possible from the staff in order to get a plan adopted. In most situations, a health and fitness manager who attempts to play a lone hand in getting a plan approved will find the going really rough. It is much better to use all the staff, if available, in any planning effort.

10. *Divide and rule:* This approach endeavors to weaken the opposition to a plan by creating a split within its members. In some situations this strategy has been successful, although it does have its drawbacks. It does suppress cooperative efforts among the staff and it has a tendency to impede dynamic leadership.[12]

MAJOR ELEMENTS OF STRATEGIC HEALTH AND FITNESS PROGRAM PLANNING

Four major elements are essential in the appraisal stage of strategic health and fitness program planning. These include an analysis of

---

12. Adapted from Terry and Franklin, *Principles,* pp. 159–161.

(1) the program's mission, (2) the organization, (3) the manager's values, and (4) the program's strengths and weaknesses.

Analysis of Mission:
What is the Program's Purpose?

The main purpose of an organization's health and fitness program is to promote the total health of its participants—physically, mentally and emotionally. The program must be designed in such a way as to attract these individuals so that they, in turn, build a strong attachment to the program.

A secondary purpose is to affect health-enhancing life-styles through programs of health education and fitness. These programs, if presented in a professional manner, can have a positive effect on their participants. A good program helps employees make choices which can result in living more healthful and happy lives. An important point to remember, however, is that changing an individual's behavior is difficult.

Analysis of the Organization:
Who are These Potential Participants?

People interested in health and fitness (executives of corporations included) are potential participants in a well-planned program. Both a health and fitness interest survey and a health and fitness needs survey should precede the implementation of any component. An analysis of the results of both these surveys will provide valuable data prior to designing the comprehensive program. But only after the data of the two surveys have been analyzed should any of the components be initiated. The program must center upon the health awareness of all participants. No one will argue that people are the most valuable resource of any organization; therefore, the program must focus upon them. The major goal, then, is to strive to have as many potential participants as possible enroll in health education programs and/or fitness programs or both and actively participate regardless of age, sex, physical condition, or present life-style.

Analysis of the Manager's Values:
Where Do the Manager's Values Come From?

Values that affect a manager's behavior and are considered good or bad, important or unimportant, are derived from three sources: the individual, the program, and the organization. They serve as a means or standard for evaluating things, events, activities, and programs; therefore, they help these managers deal with their environments. Values are especially useful in comparing decision alternatives, since the alternatives can be compared against values.

Since values develop primarily from the background of the manager, they influence their desires and plans. Three factors that influence the background values of managers are education, religion, and ethics.

Values can also evolve from the health and fitness program. The manager's assessment of the program as to its fair, good, or high quality can be viewed as placing a set of values on it. Naturally, all managers aspire to conduct high-quality programs and to succeed, but there have been and will be failures.

The values assigned to the organization by the managers are influenced by (1) perceptions of the organization and problems encountered, (2) decisions and solutions to problems, (3) interpersonal relationship with employees and top management, (4) effect of pressures and stress, and (5) organizational success.

> Owners of health and fitness organizations control many important processes, for example, the reward system, recruitment, selection, and promotion. Owners should use these processes to shape the implementation of strategy in the organization. One important way of doing this is to select only those managers whose values are congruent with those of the organization and its owners.[13]

Analysis of the Program: What Are Its Strengths and Weaknesses?

An internal evaluation of a health and fitness program can identify its strengths and weaknesses. Morale and motivation, however, are two factors which may be very difficult to measure; therefore, managers should be careful in making too positive claims of success. A well-planned program monitors participants over a specified time period to determine success rates. However, this evaluation is conducted at the site

---

13. Voyer, personal communication.

and is frequently limited to tracking participants. What cannot be evaluated is what, if any, behavior modifications or life-style changes participants have made that can be attributed to the program.

When health and fitness programs are implemented, they may be strong in delivering health education programs and weak in offering fitness programs or vice versa. Through the evaluation process, weaknesses can be detected and then corrected. However, funds, trained personnel, facilities, and equipment are all necessary in order to strengthen weak programs.

TACTICAL PLANNING

Earlier in this chapter, the word "strategy" was defined as it is commonly used in the military and in the field of management. The word "tactic," also derived from military usage, describes the arranging and maneuvering of military and naval personnel. In management usage, tactics are used in short-range planning for the allocating of resources and for the scheduling of actual tasks that must be accomplished within a short period of time. Furthermore, tactical plans are more specified, detailed, and difficult to change once they have been implemented than are strategic plans. Strategic plans, on the other hand, establish a basic structure wherein tactical plans may be implemented. It should be noted here that tactical plans are the same as operational plans.

With regard to health and fitness programming, tactical planning answers the question: How do we get there? When long-range programs goals are broken down into short-range plans, the manager can more clearly see the direction of the program in day-to-day activities and can assure that these activities are contributing to the long-range goals. In other words, working toward more immediate and more tangible goals provides the manager a way of relieving the frustration that can occur from difficulty of accomplishing a major long-range goal. Tactical plans provide a means of measuring progress and exercising control over the program. As each tactical plan is achieved, the results can be evaluated and any necessary adjustments to the long-range goals can be made.[14]

The budget for a comprehensive health and fitness program is one of the best examples of tactical planning. It must be precise and is usually

---

14. Adapted from Harvey Kahalas, "Planning Types and Approaches: A Necessary Function," *Managerial Planning*, 28:6, 23, May/June, 1980.

planned for one fiscal year. If a program is comprehensive, then, of course, the budget must reflect all its components or programs. This is to say that all components will operate under the one budget. But, on the other hand, it is conceivable that each component has its own budget and must operate its program within the overall budget. (More information on budgets may be found in Chapter XI.)

DIFFERENCES BETWEEN GOALS AND OBJECTIVES

An integral part of an effective planning process is establishing goals and objectives. Planning should involve all health and fitness personnel and the manager so that both short-term and long-term plans may be formulated. When goals and objectives are clearly defined, a definitive description of needs and services is possible.

There are differences between goals and objectives. Goals are general statements of purpose. They are expressed in terms of desired results or outcomes, indicating the reasons why programs are conducted. Usually, goals are achieved over a long period of time, extending anywhere from one year to five years. As part of the planning process, they should be viewed annually but not necessarily changed. A goal is analogous to a high-rise building, in that there are many steps before a desired floor is reached.

Just as each floor reached indicates progress, so objectives serve as indices as to how much has been accomplished. Objectives are statements that are measurable, observable behavior that lead toward a goal. Whereas goals have an indeterminate life span, objectives define time limits precisely. Objectives lend concrete reality to rather vague hopes that are often contained in goal statements. They allow participants to define experiences that can measurably determine whether there is movement toward a goal. A well-stated objective will provide specific guidelines for participant, instructor, manager, program, and organization and will clarify what each of these must do to reach desired goals. There are both goals and objectives for the participants, the instructor, the manager, the program, and the organization. The selection of the goals and objectives should always be in accordance with the capabilities of the participant, the instructor, and the manager as well as the availability of resources within the organization.

SETTING GOALS:
AN OPPORTUNITY FOR CREATIVE THINKING

The major goal of a comprehensive health and fitness program is to affect the mental and physical well-being of participants, whereas the primary motive of developing and implementing such a program is to assist the organization in the attainment of its goals. The major program goal and the major goals of an organization are interrelated.

All organizations, regardless of their size and mission, have set goals they wish to attain; but placed in priority, the one major goal is to have all employees acquire and practice good health and fitness habits. Clearly, without healthy people, organizations cannot adequately function to provide a product or service. Health and fitness programs, too, have goals they hope to accomplish; but again at the top of the list is the goal to have participants learn and practice holistic health.

The day-to-day tasks involved in organizing and administering a health and fitness program leave little time for thinking ahead to determine what needs to be accomplished. Goals that seem to be unrealistic at present may become real possibilities in the future. Goal setting can release the creative energies of both instructors and managers; therefore, effective planning can translate into reality.

Health and fitness instructors support goals that reflect their creative thinking. If goal setting does not bring about the hopes and desires of the staff, the end product will be only definitions of what is already being done. Goals will move participants to a higher level of functioning and instructors, managers, and programs to a higher level of effectiveness.

One approach to stimulate visionary thinking might be as follows:

- Prepare the instructional staff for a few sessions in creative thinking and have their permission to engage in brainstorming as a group.
- Tell the staff to relax so that they do not feel pressured.
- Ask the question, What could be happening at our organization or at a particular organization one year from now if really positive changes occur?
- Ask the staff to visualize concrete events that could happen. They should be specific about what they foresee happening among the participants, instructors, and the program.
- Have the members list the images that they perceive individually, then share them with the entire staff.

- Write all the ideas on a large white easel pad so that all may see.
- Identify the concepts that seem to be similar or in the same general area. Have the staff select at least four or five concepts that could be translated into goals.

Steps for Defining Goals

Although many goals are implicit as they relate to participants, instructors, managers and programs, the selection of a few explicit, commonly held goals helps to focus energies, exercise creative behavior, and develop imagination. Goals provide a challenge to see beyond current demands and identify the values inherent in them. Once the instructors and the manager agree to meet a few times, they can clarify goals and create a future-oriented climate within the staff.

There are six specific steps that may be utilized when defining goals:

- Several meetings must be held which all health and fitness instructors are required to attend. Furthermore, any interested employees should attend.
- At these meetings, each staff person must come up with a list of items that are to be written on large white easel pads. An "S" is placed beside items that are similar or quite similar; and "R" is placed beside items that refer to the same issue; a "G" is placed beside items that fall into the same general area.
- For the purpose of clarity, each staff person attending the meetings may ask questions of other persons. The manager then goes through the complete list with all members to note which of the items are similar to others and to what degree.
- The group then identifies those items that are most common. These are listed on another page in summary form that is agreed to by the staff.
- After listing the four or five issues that are most common, they are rank-ordered by the staff, through discussion, in terms of the greatest importance.
- The issues are refined and restated as goals.

DEVELOPING GOOD OBJECTIVES

When determining objectives, one should ask the following questions:

- What observations will show that progress is being made toward a goal?

- What observations will show that there is digression from a goal?
- What can be done within the capabilities of the participants, the instructor, the skills of the manager, and the resources available for the program to reach a goal?

Poor objectives can lead to confusion and undermine a staff's intention to accomplish a goal. A poor objective tends to increase ambiguity rather than reduce it.

A good objective considers four questions:

- What will be accomplished?
- Who and what will be measured?
- When will the measurement take place?
- How much progress toward the standard has been reached?

"What" refers to the action to be completed; "who" and "what" refer to the participants, the instructors, the manager and the program; "when" refers to a specific date; and "how much" refers to some standard or quality to be achieved.

Steps for Defining Objectives

- After the staff have agreed on four or five goal statements, they should now focus on one goal at a time.
- The staff must ask the question, What objectives must be accomplished if this goal is to be reached? There will be many answers, and they should be written on a large white easel pad.
- After completing the previous step, the members look at the variety of answers and select several of them, using the following criteria:

    Is this an important change?
    Is it measurable?
    Can it be observed in some way?
    Is it an indicator of the goal?

- The small list that results from the previous step will become the *what* of one or more objectives. At this time the staff should begin to identify the *who* and *what* for which the objective is defined.
- Now the *when* should be considered. It may be reasonable to define a target date at this time. It is often more useful, however, to delay setting a target date until objectives are clarified in order to allow enough time for everything to get done.

- Defining the *how much* part of the progress toward an objective may involve expert advice on evaluation. It also means that the staff must reach a consensus on reasonable expectations from the participant, the instructor, and the program. The following procedures may prove helpful:
- Brainstorm ideas about evaluations and expectations. These ideas should be written down.
- Select some staff member or hire a consultant who is familiar with evaluation and measurement to work with the group.
- Define and reword the ideas, clarify measurement procedures and expectations, and have the group discuss the well-formed objectives at another meeting.
- When objectives are completed and agreed upon, review all of the objectives for clarity and reasonableness, make any adjustments that are necessary.

What is known as the process of management by goals and objectives (MBGO) has just been discussed. MBGO is commonly referred to as a planning technique in which managers and their staffs jointly develop goals and objectives. MBGO also serves as a motivational technique, since its goals and objectives setting, participation, and feedback components can enhance motivation.

Management by goals and objectives fits perfectly both the purpose and style of a health and fitness program. It clarifies goals, makes objectives better understandable, increases commitment, and achieves good results, thus mutually benefiting the participant, the instructor, the manager, the program, and the organization.

SUGGESTED GOALS AND OBJECTIVES

For the participant, the instructor, the manager, the program, and the organization there are suggested goals and objectives. For purposes of clarity, health education and fitness are separate; yet, a comprehensive program must include both. The manager is of prime importance in developing and implementing these goals and objectives.

Health Education Goals and Objectives

	Goals	*Objectives*
Participant	To understand the basic facts concerning health, disease, and nutrition	To participate in a variety of health education offerings from the program
		To keep oneself informed through reading, TV, radio, and so forth on nutrition, health risk diseases, and stress-related illnesses, and on what can be done to prevent and manage them
	To evaluate present health practices	To carry out a personal health risk assessment
		To identify needed changes
		To follow up on any problems with the physician
	To incorporate health enhancing life-style changes into daily routine.	To have a complete physical examination annually
		To stop smoking immedately
		To reduce consumption of chemical substances immediately
		To improve diet immediately
		To begin a safe weight-loss routine immediately.
Instructor	To obtain more knowledge about, and to stay current on, health-related issues in order to teach others effectively	To attend workshops, symposia, or conferences on heealth, disease, and nutrition on a regular basis
		To read regularly about health-related issues
	To obtain more knowledge about how to assist participants to evaluate thoroughly and modify their health practices and their needs.	To improve health interviewing skills through training and practice
		To improve health assessment techniques through training and practice
		To improve health counseling techniques through training and practice
		To develop expertise in record-keeping methods through training and experimentation.

Manager	To gain an understanding of the fundamentals of health education management in an organization	To acquire better management skills through workshops, conferences, and reading
		To acquire a better understanding and more complete knowledge of health issues by reading and attending conferences
		To learn about computerized information management and to apply it to health program management
	To gain an understanding about, and to implement, a health education program that will provide maximum benefits to participants.	To research the needed components of a health education program
		To develop staff training procedures
		To develop and update written program protocols, policies, and procedures
		To develop and implement assessment, interview, counseling, and teaching tools.
Program	To produce health-enhancing life-style changes through education of participants	To provide information which participants more aware of health risk diseases, stress-related illnesses, and information about what can be done to prevent or manage such diseases
		To develop and implement personal health assessment packages
	To expand and diversify program offerings to meet changing needs of participants	To expand the number of health education offerings to include topics such as cancer, pregnancy, arthritis, stroke, and mental health
		To list guidelines to be used for each health education offering
	To develop standards for each health program offered.	To research standards that are recommended by accrediting agencies, if available

		To adopt/modify standards to fit one's own program
		To evaluate the program regularly.
Organization	To promote the health of employees and their families	To supply participants regularly with written information about health education programs
		To inform all new participants about the program(s)
		To develop policies that permit/ encourage participation
	To improve the working environment	To conduct a health risk appraisal and correct potential hazards in the organization within a specified time
		To provide employees with all health risk information pertaining to specific jobs
		To post safety risks and health hazard notices where applicable.
	*To improve productivity	
	*To reduce medical benefits usage	
	*To reduce human resource management costs	It is in the interest of the organization to develop routine ways to monitor:
	*To improve public image of the organization.	• Turnover rates • Absenteeism • Grievances/complaints • Morale • Medical benefits usage • Internal/external image.

---

*These four goals are the primary reasons for the organization's support of employee health education programs.

Fitness Goals and Objectives

	Goals	*Objectives*
Participant	To improve flexibility	To understand the value and benefits of being physically fit
	To increase aerobic capacity or cardio-vascular endurance	To participate in a regular fitness program of calisthenics, aerobics, cool-downs, and relaxation exercises
	To improve muscular endurance To improve muscular strength	To participate in a regular fitness program of weight training To evaluate progress and incorporate changes into personal program when appropriate
	To improve physical appearance	To attend program-sponsored activities regularly
	To improve mental attitude	To encourage family members to participate regularly in programs and activities
	To alleviate lower back pain, leg pain, muscle aches, and so forth	
	To increase the amount and variety of par-ticipation in fitness programs by oneself and one's family.	
Instructor	To obtain specific knowledge in the area of fitness instructional methods including calisthenics, aerobics, weight training and relaxation exercises	To participate in work-shops, seminars and so forth and to read books and and periodicals about methods of teaching calisthenics, aerobics, weight training and relaxation exercises
	To obtain more knowl-edge about how to assist participants to evaluate thoroughly and modify their fitness practices	To improve fitness interviewing skills through training and practice To improve fitness counseling techniques through training and practice

		To improve fitness assessment and screening techniques through training and practice
		To experiment with different instructional methods to see which work best
		To develop expertise in record-keeping methods through training and experimentation.
Manager	To gain an understanding about, and to carry out, the fundamentals of managing fitness program(s)	To research the desired components of a comprehensive fitness program
		To develop and update written program protocol, policies, and procedures, including one's own confidentiality
	To gain an understanding about, and carry out, a comprehensive marketing strategy	To develop staff training procedures
		To develop and implement assessment, interview, counseling and teaching tools
		To develop a computerized individualized fitness evaluation process
		To develop evaluation strategies
		To research similar programs used to market their activities
		To develop a marketing strategy that fits the resources and goals of the program.
Program	To promote health-enhancing life-style changes through programs of fitness	To provide information about and encourage participation in fitness
		To develop and implement personal fitness assessment and screening
	To expand and diversify program offerings to meet changing needs of participants	To provide a continuum of components which addresses a varity of interests as well as a variety of fitness needs

	To develop standards for each fitness component offered.	To assess continually changing needs
		To research standards that are recommended by accrediting agencies, if available
		To modify/adopt appropriate standards to fit one's own program.
Organization	To unify employees through fitness activities.	To provide components which could reach individuals who prefer group participation as well as those who prefer individual participation
		To design the program so as to encourage participation in some activities by participants' families
		To design programs which afford opportunities for interpersonal communication
		To publish a monthly fitness newsletter for employees.*

SUMMARY

It is one of the manager's major roles to establish a continuous planning process. Successful health and fitness programs, as does any program, require good planning. A manager must plan carefully in order for program implementation to be effective, usually relying on staff personnel to assist in the planning process. Proper timing, sufficient funding, and adequate facilities are essential to the planning of programs. Short, intermediate, or long-range plans will dictate the time spans. Single-use plans, or plans created for one situation, and standing-use plans, the guidelines for the program, are the two types of plans the manager uses to achieve goals and objectives.

Managers of health and fitness programs have many responsibilities, one of which is program planning. This latter task is extremely important in order to arouse and sustain the interest of participants.

Strategic planning can be a helpful process in achieving effective

---

*Note other organizational goals and objectives under "Health Education" section.

management. A manager cannot foresee changes in technology, society, future impacts of decisions, or the increased pressures of competition. Therefore, planning strategies should be devised somehow to prepare the manager for such unforeseen occurrences.

Steps in strategy planning include identifying specific goals and objectives and developing a program to focus on these goals and objectives, structuring the program, employing competent staff members, and evaluating the various steps taken.

As pertaining to health and fitness programs, planning goes through analysis stages which include deciding the manager's values, the purpose of the program, participants in the program, and the program's strengths and weaknesses. All these factors should be defined and analyzed.

Short-range planning for allocating resources and scheduling tasks is known as tactical planning. This type of planning involves specifics and details in order to see clearly how the program is functioning and to spot flaws which should be corrected.

Goals and objectives need to be separately defined. Goals tend to be generally stated in broad terms and have an indeterminate life span. Objectives, on the other hand, are measurable behaviors having a definite time and leading toward a goal. Both goals and objectives are necessities in effective planning.

One method which works well in the attainment of goals and objectives is management by goals and objectives (MBGO). MBGO clarifies goals and objectives, increases commitment, and achieves results.

The chapter culminates with a listing of suggested goals and objectives for the participant, the instructor, the manager, the program, and the organization. In all of this planning, the manager's role is vital.

Chapter IV

PLANNING THE HEALTH AND FITNESS PROGRAM: DESIGN, CONTENT AND RELATED CONSIDERATIONS

DESIGNING THE COMPREHENSIVE PROGRAM

One of the most important tasks managers are confronted with is the designing of a comprehensive health and fitness program. While some managers may have some of the necessary knowledge, others may lack it entirely. The intent of this section, then, is to present the basic steps on designing programs in hopes that both experienced and novice managers will find the information helpful.

Managers should keep in mind the fact that programs can include prevention, intervention, and rehabilitation and that a comprehensive program must include both health education programs and fitness programs. Furthermore, it is imperative that each health education component and each fitness component be carefully designed prior to being offered.

If the organization has a union(s), managers should get approval from top management before asking the leader(s) of the union(s) for ideas concerning program design. By so doing, a good working relationship will be established between management and the union(s).

The following steps are recommended for designing a comprehensive health and fitness program:

Step 1. Determine the Program Concept

Sooner or later most organizations will come to the realization that a comprehensive health and fitness program can benefit both their employees and themselves. Although most organizations have a vaguely defined idea of the purpose or mission of a health and fitness program, they do not have a program. However, they have taken the first step; for at this stage, it is not necessary for the program idea to be clearly defined.

Step 2. Conduct an Interest Survey

Some organizations feel it is prudent to conduct an interest survey prior to conducting a health and fitness needs survey. An interest survey can be useful and is taken with the assumption that employees would like to learn more about health and fitness. Furthermore, it is an acceptable statistical method of gathering information. Managers will find that interest surveys are managerially feasible and also effective for finding out the level of interest in programs that may be offered.

The information collected from a health and fitness interest survey can be utilized by managers to make predictions about enrollments in programs, to set up priorities for program offerings, and to determine the most appropriate times to schedule both health and fitness classes. A word of caution is necessary regarding enrollments in programs: These figures may not be entirely accurate because of personal factors such as change of work schedules, school calendars, fatigue, sickness, accidents, vacation periods and family obligations.

Step 3. Conduct a Needs Survey

If the results of the interest survey indicate that employees do wish to increase their knowledge about health and fitness, then a health and fitness needs survey should be conducted. Based on the results, planning components should begin. However, support from both management and the union(s), if present, is essential.

No organization will offer any kind of program unless there is a real need. A health and fitness program is worthless unless it meets the health and fitness needs of all employees.

The manager may use the following methods to survey the need for a health and fitness program:

- Collect information and pertinent data on the health and fitness needs from all employees
- Survey the employees to determine what specific health and fitness components should be offered within the comprehensive framework
- Survey management and union(s), if present, to determine what health and fitness programs they would like to see offered
- Survey other programs of comparable size, to determine what health and fitness programs they offer.

Step 4. Select an Advisory Committee

This committee should be composed of representatives from all three levels of management—top, middle, and low. An employee from each department and a union representative, if present, completes the advisory committee with the exception of a physician, who must be included either as an employee or hired as a consultant. It is of utmost importance to have complete management, union(s), if present, and employee involvement.

Step 5. Develop Goals and Objectives for the Program

Organizations that are interested in offering their employees a health and fitness program should begin by asking the basic question, What are the benefits to be derived from such a program? Management and union(s), if present, may answer the question by stating that it expects that the program will improve productivity, lessen absenteeism, increase the health knowledge and the fitness level among employees, be available to *all* employees and not just those who are high risk, and be cost effective in the long run.

After the reasons for starting a comprehensive program have been finalized, the next course of action is to develop written goals and objectives. This process may be time consuming, but it must be done if the program is to succeed.

Step 6. Increase the Level of Health Awareness

Health awareness implies having knowledge of one's health habits and the risk of illness caused by poor health practices. Andrew J.J. Brennan, director of Metropolitan Life Insurance Company's Center for Health Help, reveals:

> An employee health awareness program focuses on recognized lifestyle health risks, self-help strategies to maintain good health, and when and how to seek cost-effective health care services. By increasing health awareness, you create a favorable climate to positively influence health behaviors and patterns of using medical benefits. . . . [15]

He continues:

A number of communications vehicles can be used to convey health awareness messages such as:

---

15. Andrew J.J. Brennan, "How to Set Up a Corporate Wellness Program," *Management Review*, 72:5, 43, May, 1983.

- Health awareness newsletter . . .
- Posters and audio-visuals . . .
- Feature articles . . .
- Pamphlets . . .
- Literature racks . . .
- Guest speakers . . .

If employees are to become wise consumers of health care services it is important to educate them about their roles as active decision-makers in terms of their own and their families' health care. . . . [16]

Step 7. Identify the Resources Necessary To Implement the Program

- Determine the size and skills of the staff needed to offer the program.
- Determine what resources are available to support the program, such as office supplies, printing service, interorganizational communication system, computer facilities, postal service, and so forth.
- Determine what facilities are needed and what facilities are presently available.
- Determine what supplies and equipment are required.

Step 8. Implement the Program

After the program design has been completed, it should be rechecked. Is the design completed? Is the program design what is wanted and needed? Are all the components ready to be offered when needed? Is it necessary to make any changes so as to insure implementation?

After all the above questions have been answered, the program design is transformed into an operational program. It is impossible to determine the length of time it will take to implement any of the health education components and the fitness components, as there are several factors which influence implementation, such as costs, staff, facilities, equipment, and so forth.

Step 9. Monitor the Program's Impact

The program design should be used as a guide during implementation. But what is of vital importance is that the program be monitored so as to track its progress through a collection of data and information. The monitoring should be done periodically, depending upon the type of program being presented. For example, a four-week smoking-cessation

---

16. Ibid., pp. 43–44.

program may be monitored weekly, while a ten-week walk-jog program may be monitored every two weeks. This kind of periodic review will indicate how well the program is progressing and will clearly indicate if any changes are called for in the goals, objectives, or methods of instruction. When each health education and fitness program has been completed, a determination can be made as to whether or not the intended results have been achieved. Obviously, if the program continues, the same periodic review must also be carried out. Moreover, by monitoring programs, managers will be able to determine whether or not the original program design was satisfactory.

Step 10. Evaluate the Program

Evaluation is an integral part of program design, and it should be noted here that each component offered as well as the comprehensive program itself must be evaluated. The main purpose of evaluation is to determine whether or not the program goals and objectives are being met. In addition, the information and data gathered can be communicated to participants, thus helping them to make decisions about risk reduction and life-style changes. Finally, there are several designs managers can use for evaluating the program. "Your decision must take into account not only the limitations of any design but also the practical, ethical, and financial constraints that influence the way you conduct your evaluation."[17]

PROGRAM CONTENT

No book on management of health and fitness programs would be complete unless it contained at least a general description of potential program offerings within a comprehensive program. This section of the chapter is written with the assumption that managers are now familiar with the steps leading to the designing of a comprehensive health and fitness program.

The question that arises most frequently is, What does a manager actually need to know about the contents of a health and fitness program? At the very least, the manager should have a general working knowledge of all health and fitness components. Also, the manager's educational

---

17. Rebecca S. Parkinson and Associates, *Managing Health Promotion in the Workplace* (Palo Alto, CA: Mayfield Publishing Co., 1982), p. 47. Note: For an in-depth treatment on evaluation, see Chapter XI.

background and experience in either of these disciplines must be considered, as often he or she is called upon to be an instructor. In addition, the goals and objectives of a comprehensive program, as well as those of the organization, should be clearly understood.

There is general agreement that there are at least five major health education programs and the possibility of ten fitness programs which may be offered to employees of any organization. The number of programs offered is predicated on the size of the organization, funds, staff, equipment, and facility availability. The following are brief descriptions of the content of health and fitness programs.

HEALTH EDUCATION PROGRAMS

Environmental Management

The most basic, as well as the most important, aspect of any health education program in industry is safety. Without a safe workplace, any effort at improving employees' health will be undermined. For example, no stress-management workshop can be effective if the basic problem of noise level is not remedied.

Environmental management and safety are best handled by a team of experts consisting of an occupational health nurse, an industrial hygienist, and a safety officer. Each expert plays an integral role in identifying environmental health hazards, planning strategies to minimize the effects of these hazards, and monitoring or evaluating the impact of existing hazards if they cannot be eradicated.

Environmental hazards include noise, chemical hazards, and physical hazards. They exist in different forms and intensities depending on the specific industry. Noise levels vary but generally cause some environmental concern in every work place. The effects of noise range from individual irritation at a type of music being played to shattering vibrations requiring hearing protection. Chemical hazards demand a knowledge of the toxicology of specific hazards as well as knowledge of the routes of exposure, i.e., inhalation, absorption, or ingestion. Physical hazards such as lack of guardrails, slippery floors, heat stress, and ventilation are also problems.

Dealing with these hazards is an ongoing process. Environment is never static but varies from day to day in its effect on workers' health.

Depending on the specific hazards identified, a team of experts is necessary to deal most effectively with them. The coordination of a safe environment allows individuals the free pursuit of health without restriction in the work place setting.

Nutrition and Weight Management

Nutrition is a process of interrelated steps whereby the body assimilates food and uses it for growth and development. Nourishment is provided to the body through a diet, a pattern of eating and drinking. There is an increasing amount of evidence linking proper nutrition to health and well-being. Poor nutritional habits can increase a person's risk of hypertension, heart disease, stroke, and some forms of cancer.

Weight management is a process whereby sound dietary practices and regular physical activity maintain ideal weight. Some organizations seem to prefer to offer nutrition and weight management as two distinct separate health education programs. But because the two are interrelated, it is recommended that they be offered as one.

Managers again will have to decide who can deliver this type of program. Providers for a nutrition and weight management program may be nutritionists, dieticians, health educators, consultants, vendors, or commercial organizations, such as Weight Watchers.

Smoking Cessation

Tobacco smoking, the country's number one health problem, is also the most preventable. Diseases caused by smoking or associated with smoking are bronchitis, emphysema, arteriosclerosis, heart attacks, strokes, and cancer of the lungs, throat, mouth, larynx and pancreas.

Smoking-cessation programs should require that providers, regardless of who they are, have a basic knowledge of anatomy and physiology. They also need to be well versed in the physiology of tobacco smoking and, more specifically, in the entire smoking cycle. Organizations that are ready to offer smoking-cessation programs have options as to the provider, including a trained staff member. Naturally, there are advantages and disadvantages to each of these options depending upon the size of the organization, its goals and available resources, both human and financial.

For some employees who wish to stop smoking but have been unsuccessful, a group smoking-cessation program or a behavior modification program may be the answer. It is the prudent manager who explores all program options, as there are many different ways by which people have stopped smoking.

Stress Management

A stress management program is fundamental to any health education effort. It is important for the provider, sometimes a trained psychologist, to understand that by far the greater part of excessive stress in an employee's life is self-initiated and self-propagated. It is the employee who interprets an otherwise neutral stimulus as possessing stress-evoking characteristics. The employee reacts to the environment in accordance to his or her interpretations of the environmental stimuli. Some of the causes of stress in the work place are job changes (including promotion or demotion), new management, and a perceived lack of work skills.

Stress management programs are witnessing phenomenal growth, especially in the work place. Health and fitness managers have recognized that excessive stress that is poorly handled can have a profound negative effect on the health and job performances of employees. Managers have come to realize that there are many different approaches to stress management, such as communication skills training, supervisory training, job sharing, flex time, provision of child care, fitness activities, biofeedback, and relaxation activities. In addition to a psychologist, other trained professionals such as counselors, physical therapists, social workers, or a trained staff health educator can effectively offer a stress management program.

If stress management programs are to be successful, they must include three types of strategies for change: individual, environmental, and organizational. All three of these strategies must be put into action as a single unit if programs are to be effective.

Substance Abuse: Alcohol and Drugs

The personal abuse of alcohol and drugs, especially in the work place, has become one of the major problems facing many organizations. Chemical-dependency problems are usually caused by either poor physical or mental health, disruptive family life, financial difficulties, or the job itself. Because an employee's alcohol or drug addiction affects his or her job performance, the employee, the organization, and the union must share the problem until it is cleared up.

What are the characteristics of employees who have an alcohol or drug problem? They are usually late for work, take extended lunch hours, leave work early, miss deadlines, redo work, are continuously away from their desks or stations, are not able to concentrate, are less productive in their work than are other employees, and produce work of inferior quality.

How does an organization go about identifying employees who have a dependency on alcohol or drugs? Observation is the oldest method of screening alcohol or drug abusers in the work place and is still very effective.

What are the options open to organizations that need to choose an alcohol and drug program for their employees? The choice is predicated on the size, type of work, financial status, and union involvement of the organization. More than likely, the choice will be an employee assistance program (EAP), a program which provides professional assistance to employees who are experiencing alcohol, drug, mental, family, legal or a combination of these problems which interfere with their work performance. Most EAP programs are commonly referred to as "Broad Brush Programs" and are referral rather than treatment programs. Often, organizations will help train staff, supervisors, or union officials to detect problems. These leaders can become skilled enough to recognize problems and make the proper referral to the EAP. Sometimes, an organization will hire a professional consultant to develop and implement an EAP. Most organizations do not have a person on the staff with the expertise and experience necessary to assist in program design.

Another option can be the consortium approach. This approach calls for two or more organizations that pool human and financial resources and share the responsibilities of assisting employees who have alcohol or drug problems.

INTRODUCTION TO FITNESS PROGRAMS

Although managers may or may not become involved with instruction, it seems advisable to provide them with some background information in the area of fitness. Since fitness programs are based on physical or health-related components, it seems only logical to define each of these components. Furthermore, this section will also take up the principles of exercise, define each of the kinds of exercises, and briefly describe the seven regular fitness programs and the three rehabilitation fitness programs.

Physical or Health-Related Fitness Components

Following are definitions of the five physical or health-related fitness components:

- Cardiovascular endurance—the capacity to sustain vigorous physical activity, 20 to 30 minutes or longer, that will increase the supply of oxygen to the heart, lungs and vascular system
- Muscle strength—the capacity of a muscle to exert a maximal force against resistance
- Muscle endurance—the capacity of a muscle to exert a force repeatedly over a period of time or to apply strength and sustain it
- Flexibility—a measure of the range of motion performed without undue stress to a joint or a group of joints
- Body fat composition—the percentage of body weight which is fat.

Principles of Exercise

Briefly discussed below are the principles of exercise:

- Frequency—How often should people exercise? Initially, a good physical fitness program will require that the individual work out three or four times per week. The participant should keep in mind that fitness cannot be stored; it must be renewed continuously. Each exercise session requires the proper intensity and duration. Most people, if they adhere to the principle of frequency, will discover that improvements can be realized in between ten to twelve weeks.
- Intensity—The degree of difficulty is the key for cardiovascular and muscular strength and endurance improvement. With respect to cardiovascular fitness, target heart rate is related to energy cost; and it serves as an excellent tool for measurement. The proper intensity may be calculated in two ways. First, the formula 220 minus the person's age; second, the Karvonen formula, which is 60–80 percent

of the difference between the resting and maximal heart rates. However, researchers now claim that 75–85 percent of the difference between the resting and maximal heart rates is safe and gives both training effect and a method for monitoring activity levels. A quick pulse rate will indicate exercise rate if the pace has been continuous.

• Duration—is interrelated with intensity. In order to produce the required cardiovascular results, a specified amount of time is needed. At least 20 to 30 minutes of continuous physical activity are required to achieve cardiovascular benefits. If the duration of the exercise does not meet the time requirements, overloading is not sufficient to produce changes.

• Mode of Activity—When an activity is selected, the individual should know what benefits are derived when it is performed regularly. Activities that produce good cardiovascular fitness are vigorous, continuous, and rhythmic; and they utilize the total body, for example, running, walking, swimming, skiing. Heart rate response is the key to these types of activities. On the other hand, if muscular strength and muscular endurance are desired, weight training and timed calisthenics are the types of activities that should be performed.

• Overload—In order for one's body to improve, one must perform more work than he or she is normally accustomed to. The more conditioned people become, the harder it is for them to reach their target heart rates. Therefore, "overloading" is necessary in all fitness and physical conditioning programs. Gradually increasing the work load over a period of time will result in improved cardiovascular endurance or muscular strength and endurance predicated on the kind of fitness program undertaken. Overloading can be accomplished in two ways: by increasing the *total work*, i.e., run further or play longer, and/or by increasing the *work rate*, i.e., run faster or play harder. With highly unconditioned individuals, overloading should be prescribed in small increments.

• Progression—If one's body is to show improvement, one must be exposed to more and more intense levels of exercise. This advancement can be accomplished by the use of both overload and progression, as they are similar in nature. If a person stays at one particular fitness level, physiological adaptation takes place. This level is fine for fitness maintenance but not for advancement for beginners or improved performance for athletes.

• Specificity—The body responds differently to different activities imposed upon it. Thus, fitness improvements are specific to special training regimes. A sound fitness program can use specificity for each component:

Muscular strength and endurance results from weight training.

Flexibility is derived from stretching and relaxation exercises.

Cardiovascular endurance comes from aerobic activities.

Body composition is the product of nutritional understanding and proper eating.

Specificity can be better accomplished from regular routines and not from random exercising.

- Use or Disuse—Simply stated, *use* promotes function while *disuse* promotes deterioration. Many people often illustrate the concept of disuse. Viewing the population as a whole, one sees that, in general, they are too sedentary and should become more physically active. Inactivity leads to poor muscle tone and strength and to decalcification of bones. X-rays of bones clearly demonstrate this decalcification in persons who are non-weight bearing. A similar x-ray finding is evident in those individuals who have a cast applied for a fractured leg, for example, and are immobile over a period of time. Therefore, weight bearing should be reestablished as soon as possible and active exercise begun as soon as clinically indicated.

- Individual Differences—People cannot be stereotyped, because human beings respond to exercise in their own way and at their own rate. This fact is especially true when one is conducting an exercise program or choosing an exercise partner. Different risk factors will have a direct bearing on each individual.

Examples:

Obesity (a major concern in exercise programs): Obese individuals usually need to lose weight first, then perhaps participate in a walk/jog program.

Lower Back Rehabilitation: Individuals need slow progression exercises specifically designed to deal with the problem.

Cardiac Rehabilitation: Individuals need certain specific kinds of exercises.

Orthopedic Rehabilitation: Individuals usually need cycling and swimming.

Injuries: Individuals need modification of program in addition to rehabilitation.

People exercise under all types of environmental conditions: extreme heat, cold, on and under water, and at various altitudes. Exercise physiologists have investigated all of these various conditions. As a result, an extensive body of knowledge is now available to people exercising under these varied conditions.

Kinds of Exercise

Following are definitions of the seven kinds of exercise:

- Aerobics (with oxygen)—any exercise that is vigorous and prolonged, 20–30 minutes or more, which supplies oxygen to the body through the cardiorespiratory system
- Anaerobics (without oxygen)—any exercise that is not prolonged or sustained in which the oxygen supply to the body is insufficient
- Calisthenics—any exercise which does not involve the use of barbells and dumbbells or weight training machines. These exercises may be timed or done to music.
- Isokinetic (dynamic)—any exercise in which the muscle is able to shorten or lengthen to counteract an accommodating resistance developed by a device that allows only a constant rate of movement regardless of the force exerted by a contracting muscle
- Isometric (static)—any exercise in which the length of the muscle does not shorten during contractions, tension develops, heat is produced, but no mechanical work is performed
- Isotonic (dynamic)—any exercise in which the muscle is able to contract, shorten or lengthen, and perform work
- Progressive Resistance—any exercise used to increase muscle strength by utilizing the overload principle, i.e., subjecting the muscle to a greater-than-normal load.

FITNESS PROGRAMS
CARDIOVASCULAR ENDURANCE

All the programs described below are aimed at developing cardiovascular endurance or aerobic capacity:

Aerobic Dance

Aerobic dance is a choreographed exercise program which is concerned primarily with developing cardiovascular endurance, but it also increases muscular endurance and flexibility. Relaxation exercises are also included in an aerobic dance program. Sessions usually are organized to consist of warm-ups, aerobic conditioning, cool down, and relaxation exercises. Aerobic conditioning is accomplished through simple *dances* that range from slow, stretching warm-ups to strenuous, rhythmical routines. This workout pattern is followed by exercises performed on mats to improve muscle tone, muscle strength, and flexibility. Moreover, the development of proper body mechanics and maximum range of motion are integral parts of the program. Finally, various muscular relaxation exercises complete each session. All the above-mentioned elements, combined with music and dance, offer participants much fun, challenge, and a feeling of well-being.

Aerobic Exercise

Aerobic exercise is a comprehensive exercise program consisting of aerobic conditioning, muscular endurance and toning, postural flexibility, and relaxation. Floor *exercises* done to contemporary music make up the aerobic portion of the classes. Various relaxation techniques are utilized at the end of each class.

Aquatic Fitness

Aquatic fitness is a complete cardiovascular program for those who prefer swimming for exercise. Non-swimmers may also enroll in these types of programs, as there are a variety of non-swimming exercises which can be performed at the shallow end of a pool. Although any stroke or combination of strokes may be used, it is generally advisable to have the participants begin with the resting strokes, such as breaststroke, sidestroke, and elementary backstroke, until they become accustomed to the workout routine; then they may employ more vigorous strokes.

Each aquatic exercise class should contain three main components:

- A combination warm-up/water calisthenics routine performed in the shallow end of the pool
- A peak exercise period to elevate the heart rates to improve cardio-

vascular endurance (swimming, shallow water walking exercises, bobbing, kicking, and water games), and

- A cool-down period of slow walking and swimming and final stretch-downs on the pool deck.

Walk/Jog

Walk/jog is an exercise program designed for people who have been sedentary or who otherwise are not in good physical condition. Most of these types of programs have been based on the "Y's Way To Fitness," a nationwide program of cardiovascular endurance training.

Each class session in a typical walk/jog program consists of the resting pulse rate, warm-ups, peak workout, target pulse rate, cool down, relaxation exercises, and the post-exercise pulse rate. These programs are usually divided into ten-week sessions, and individuals start as beginners. Each class session should begin very slowly and progress gradually during each of the following weeks. After this program, the participants may wish to continue into intermediate, then advanced, programs. Instructors should be advised, moreover, that with entry into each new level of the program, participants are developing cardiovascular endurance as well as improving muscular strength and endurance.

MUSCULAR STRENGTH AND ENDURANCE

The following are designed to develop muscular strength and endurance:

Weight Training

Weight training, or progressive resistance exercise, is a program utilizing assorted weights, either barbells and dumbbells, or weight training machines, for performing exercises. A sound weight training program should follow a developmental pattern and should be programmed to meet the specific physical needs of the individual.

A basic weight training program should include most of the major muscle and muscle groups, and there should be at least three workouts a week. The participants should perform three sets (a stated number of repetitions) of exercises during the sessions and take a five-minute rest between each set. Each exercise should be performed eight to ten repetitions (going through the full exercise one time). The amount of weight used depends on the physical status of the participant. Beginners should always start with a light load and add weights as they progress. All exercises should be performed without straining.

Timed Calisthenics

A timed calisthenics program can be designed to help participants develop muscular strength and endurance. At every class session, the participant performs the exercises repetitiously and increases the number of exercises performed within a predetermined time interval. For example, as a beginner who is in poor physical condition, a person may perform five sit-ups in one minute. At about the second week, the same person may perform seven sit-ups in one minute and gradually increase the number until he or she is capable of performing a satisfactory number of sit-ups in a specified number of minutes.

When presenting timed calisthenics, the instructor should start with exercises for the neck and work down to the toes. In addition, exercises should be given that include the total body and body parts.

FLEXIBILITY

Static stretching exercises may be utilized to develop flexibility. Each exercise should be sustained for six to seven seconds. When these exercises are presented in a series, they compromise a program. In most instances, selected flexibility exercises, sometimes referred to as warm-ups, precede any training or workout session because it is at this time that the muscles and joints of the body need to be loosened and stretched. Many people lack overall flexibility because they do not use certain muscles and joints in their work and daily lives.

Participants should be instructed to perform the various exercises slowly and *not bounce* in an attempt to stretch further (called ballistic stretching). Gaining a satisfactory level of overall flexibility takes time and patience. For some it may be advisable to use a combination of flexibility exercises and some type of cardiovascular endurance activity.

REHABILITATION FITNESS PROGRAMS

Briefly discussed below are three types of rehabilitation fitness programs:

Cardiac Rehabilitation

Cardiac rehabilitation is a medically supervised exercise program for people who have suffered a heart attack, have experienced open-heart surgery, or may be significantly at risk of heart attacks. For these individuals, the advice and counsel of a cardiologist is essential in helping to develop the exercise prescription for the participant. Initially, a graded exercise or stress test should be administered in a medical setting: in a hospital, a clinic, or a physician's office.

The cardiac rehabilitation exercise program must have close medical supervision at each class session. The content for each class usually includes flexibility exercises and walking and/or slow jogging, and the class terminates with relaxation exercise.

All participants must be referred to a cardiac exercise program by their organization's medical department or their personal physicians. While the program provides ongoing medical supervision during each exercise session, it is not intended to replace the role of the primary physician. Throughout the program, periodic reports of progress should be provided by the organization offering a cardiac rehabilitation exercise program.

Pulmonary Rehabilitation

Pulmonary rehabilitation is an exercise program for individuals who have asthma, chronic bronchitis, emphysema, or who otherwise suffer from pulmonary insufficiency. As with the cardiac exercise program, these participants must be referred to the pulmonary exercise program by the organization's medical department or by their primary care physician.

Pulmonary programs provide opportunities for individuals to receive instruction in the anatomy and physiology of respiration, breathing exercises, relaxation exercises, respiratory hygiene, medications, and diets. The philosophy of a typical pulmonary rehabilitation exercise program is that learning should be active rather than passive and that participants are part of an involved team and are expected to share responsibility for their care. Classes and activities should be planned and organized so as to provide individuals with opportunities to learn and practice skills, integrate knowledge, and become involved in personalizing their own home programs.

Low Back Rehabilitation

Low back, a program for individuals with functional lower back problems, consists of low-level exercise routines designed to relieve stress and induce relaxation of the various muscle groups. As the exercise sessions progress, improvements in flexibility and basic muscle strength should be noticeable. The emphasis in this program is on the improvements of postural muscular strength and endurance, body flexibility, and relaxation techniques.

In addition to the low-back exercise sessions, lectures on specific topics are an integral part of the program. These topics are related to low-back problems and include such items as body anatomy and physiology, causation factors, body mechanics, and nutrition and weight control.

RELATED CONSIDERATIONS

The last section of this chapter focuses on three important considerations which are an integral part of planning a comprehensive health and fitness program. Each of the topics to be discussed plays an important role and it seems prudent that managers acquaint themselves with all three.

Scheduling Health and Fitness Classes

An issue that confronts managers is that of scheduling classes, and central to scheduling health and fitness classes for an organization's employees is accessibility and convenience. But before any class can be scheduled, a decision must be made by top management regarding the time classes can be scheduled, i.e., on the organization's time or on the employees' time. If the classes are scheduled on an organization's time, the advantages are that more employees will participate because these classes will not take away time from their families and community obligations.

The disadvantages for scheduling health and fitness classes on an organization's time are that there is less time for production, resulting in less profit and more cost; conflict with the work hours of both management and employees; and the need for permission for work release.

If classes are scheduled on employees' time, the advantages are that working hours are not interrupted, production quotas are met, and those who enroll in a program usually have made a commitment.

The disadvantages for scheduling health and fitness classes on employees' time are that many do not choose to relinquish their own time and need to rush in order to participate, many will not participate if classes are not held on site, and many will not participate if classes are held during their vacation periods.

Health education classes are often scheduled during lunchtime. If employees bring their own lunch, they may eat during the lecture. Such classes are referred to as "lunch and learn." If health classes are not held during lunchtime, they are usually held immediately after work.

If fitness classes are held on employees' time during lunch hour, employees will need time to shower. Finding the time to eat after class thus becomes a problem and some employees will skip lunch. For this reason, it may be advisable to conduct fitness classes before work or immediately after work.

Some organizations have what is known as flex-time, i.e., employees are allowed to choose their own working hours within certain limits. However, some organizations require that all employees work certain core hours, for example, from 9:00 A.M. to 2:00 P.M. Flex-time will allow employees time to attend health and fitness classes. However, flex-time is not conducive to shift work.

If on the organization's time, health education classes and fitness classes obviously can be scheduled anytime during working hours, shifts included. The hours for fitness classes, however, will depend to a large extent on the number of employees who enroll. One way to find out the most convenient hours for fitness classes is to ask for this information on an interest survey.

Planning for Fitness Classes

Whether or not managers teach exercise classes, they should know how to plan for these classes. Exercise classes, as a rule, should include participants at three fitness levels: beginning, intermediate, and advanced. It is at the beginning level that participants learn how to take their pulse rate, learn their exercise target heart rate, and learn the exercises and the routines. They must be cautioned, however, about overexertion at the beginning.

When the number of enrollees increases and the class schedule permits, each exercise class should be divided into the three fitness levels so that each participant can work out within his or her respective exercise level. The three fitness levels are briefly described as follows:

- Beginning—In most cases, all new participants start at the beginner's level. Instructors should follow a prescribed progressive series of exercises. Once an employee successfully completes the beginning program, he or she is allowed to enroll in the intermediate program.
- Intermediate—This program consists of two fitness levels: those who have successfully completed the beginning program and those who have been at the intermediate level for ten weeks or more. There is also another way to enter the intermediate program: by receiving a satisfactory score on an aerobic capacity test. Basically all participants perform the same exercises and routines, but the intermediate level has increased time and overloading. For example, beginners walk while the intermediate group jogs, or beginners walk or jog slowly and the intermediate group performs aerobic exercises.
- Advanced—This program also consists of two fitness levels: those who have successfully completed the intermediate program and those who have been at the advanced level for ten weeks or more. Another way to enter the advanced program is to score high on an aerobic capacity test. Like the beginning and intermediate programs, the advanced participants perform the same exercises and routines; the difference is the increased time or overloading for the advanced participants. Some advanced participants may not wish to remain in a structured fitness class but prefer to exercise on their own or with a friend. This is permissible as long as they perform an aerobic activity and maintain their high fitness level. Jogging, walking, swimming, tennis, racquetball, and squash are examples of good aerobic activities.

Aerobic fitness programs are usually divided into ten-week sessions: classes meet three times a week for forty-five minutes. A basic format for each class period consists of warm-ups, aerobic conditioning, calisthenics, cool down, and relaxation exercises. Beginners receive 5 to 10 minutes of aerobic conditioning at each exercise period, intermediates receive 10 to 20 minutes (overload) of aerobic conditioning, and the advanced group receive 20 to 30 minutes (overload) of aerobic conditioning. In addition, the number of repetitions for each exercise (calisthenic) increases at the last two fitness levels.

Weight training programs focusing on the development of muscular strength and muscular endurance usually are offered for four or six months; classes meet three times a week for forty-five minutes.

Factors Affecting Program Location

If a comprehensive health and fitness program is to be conducted in an organization that has departments, the program then should be located in some specific department. This issue is one that is of major concern to managers, as the location has a direct impact upon the efficiency and effectiveness of the program. In some cases, managers may have a voice in selecting a department in which to locate the program. When that is the case, careful examination of all options should be undertaken before making a decision. Because of the nature of a health and fitness program, several options are open. These options, however, are contingent upon four factors. First, how much responsibility and authority will the manager of the comprehensive program be granted? Obviously, if the manager is a novice, he or she would need more supervision than one who has experience and understands the area of management in a work place.

Second, although many organizations establish at least five major goals, when all is said and done, the bottom line is that their employees must be in good health and physically fit in order that these goals become achievable. Thus, the question arises as to what department the health and fitness program should be located in. This question is answered by Parkinson and Associates. "The most frequent locations are the medical, the benefit, and the personnel departments."[18]

A medical department is the most appropriate location for a comprehensive health and fitness program. In the absence of a medical department, it is recommended that the program be located in the human resource management department, formerly called the personnel department. The next choice is the benefits department and, lastly, the employee assistance program. Of course, there are advantages and disadvantages in locating the program in any department, but it is the department that best serves all the employees and the attitudes, atmosphere, and working

18. Parkinson and Associates, *Managing Health Promotion*, p. 26.

relationships of that particular supervising department that need to be considered in choosing a location.

The third factor is the manager's place in the chain of command. Managers of health and fitness programs must be placed high enough in the organization so as to allow them an entrance way to their immediate supervisors, not only for support and encouragement, but also to discuss problems. Moreover, managers need to have a direct line to all department heads in order to market their program and attract participants. Managers must make deciisions related to the program and must have the authority to do so. Their immediate supervisors should not become involved in any decision which has to do with the health and fitness program.

The fourth and last factor is that the department under which the program is placed must be supportive. Staff personnel working in the program must not be expected to take on additional departmental responsibilities. Moreover, the department in which the program is located tends to impact upon the success of the health and fitness program.

SUMMARY

The designing of a comprehensive health and fitness program may sound simple in theory, but actually it is quite difficult. Much thought and hard work on the part of the manager is required if the program that is designed is appropriate and meets the needs and interests of all employees. One should not attempt to design a program without first gathering information and data from both an interest survey and from a health and fitness needs survey.

Once managers acquaint themselves with the steps involved in designing a program, they also should familiarize themselves with program content. Although managers should strive to develop and implement a comprehensive health and fitness program, it is recommended that they prioritize offerings based on needs and start offerings on a small scale. Included in the program content section of this chapter are brief descriptions of five health education programs, seven regular fitness programs, and three rehabilitation fitness programs.

Health and fitness program managers will need to deal with three areas that are related to the planning process: scheduling health and fitness classes, planning for fitness classes, and program location. Each of these is discussed so that managers gain a working knowledge of all three areas in order to be better prepared to undertake the task of planning a comprehensive program. The last topic to be discussed, program location, is one in which managers may or may not have input. Nevertheless, it is important that managers understand the factors affecting program location.

Chapter V

PLANNING: SOME SUGGESTED POLICIES FOR THE HEALTH AND FITNESS PROGRAM

INTRODUCTION

As a continuation of planning, standing-use plans which include policies, procedures, and rules are discussed in this chapter. It seems feasible to devote a chapter to these three topics, with emphasis on policies, because of their importance both to managers and to health and fitness programs. For purposes of clarity, one might offer the following definitions and explanations of the words "policies," "procedures," and "rules":

Policies are essential to the efficient management of any type of organization. These are broad, comprehensive, flexible, and easy-to-interpret guidelines for making decisions and for taking action. Policies are found in most types of organizations, as they spell out the sanctioned general direction and areas to be followed. When policies are properly selected and developed, they enable each member of an organization to know what duties are to be performed, the type of performance that will result in the greatest productivity for the organization, and how best the goals and objectives can be accomplished. Thus, it is imperative that the health and fitness manager understand the organization's policies as they relate to the policies of a comprehensive health and fitness program.

Donnelly, Gibson, and Ivancevich claim that effective policies have five basic characteristics:

1. *Flexibility.* A policy must strike a reasonable balance between stability and flexibility. Conditions change, and policies must change accordingly. On the other hand, some degree of stability must prevail if order and a sense of direction are to be achieved. There are no rigid guidelines to specify the exact degree or requisite flexibility; only the judgment of management can determine the appropriate balance.

2. *Comprehensiveness.* A policy must be comprehensive to cover any contingency if plans are to be followed. The degree of compre-

hensiveness depends upon the scope of action controlled by the policy itself. If the policy is directed toward very narrow ranges of activity—for example, hiring policies—it need not be as comprehensive as a policy concerned with public relations.

3. *Coordination.* A policy must provide for coordination of various subunits whose actions are interrelated. Without coordinative direction provided by policies, each subunit is tempted to pursue its own objectives. The ultimate test of any subunit's activity should be its relationship to the policy statement.

4. *Ethical.* A policy must conform to the canons of ethical behavior which prevail in society. The manager is ultimately responsible for the resolution of issues which involve ethical principles. The increasingly complex and interdependent nature of contemporary society has resulted in a great number of problems involving ethical dimensions which are only vaguely understood.

5. *Clarity.* A policy must be written clearly and logically. It must specify the intended aim of the action which it governs, define the appropriate methods and action, and delineate the limits of freedom of action permitted to those whose actions are to be guided.[19]

Policies are developed in many ways within a program. Involvement by the full-time and part-time health and fitness staff is a most widely accepted practice. Furthermore, policies must be carefully formulated and thought out before being written. Thus, it is wise to involve the whole staff in order to look at problems affecting policies from various points of view.

Procedures are a series of related steps that are to be followed in a specific order to accomplish a given purpose. They are much more specific and narrow in scope than policies. Furthermore, policies reflect intent, whereas procedures provide ways in which plans will be carried out within the program. Therefore, new staff members need to spend a good amount of time learning proper procedures so that they can perform their duties satisfactorily.

Procedures, in order to be effective, must be formulated within the framework of policies. Therefore, it is imperative that all policies be broad in scope and clear in meaning if the formulation of procedures is to be meaningful. Managers must look at both policies and procedures as reinforcement for each other so that they can provide a considerable contribution to the achievement of established goals and objectives.

---

19. James H. Donnelly, Jr., James L. Gibson, and John M. Ivancevich, *Fundamentals of Management,* 6th ed. (Homewood, IL: Richard D. Irwin, Inc., 1987), p. 109.

The following seven points for systematic formulation of procedures should be observed by all managers:

1. A procedure should be consistent with policy statements and established objectives. Directly or indirectly, it must clearly assist in the achievement of overall goals.
2. Since environmental factors vary and internal variables are inherently different among organizations, a standard operating procedure for one organization may not be viable in another.
3. All procedures within an organization should be completely integrated and coordinated through adequate information systems.
4. People required to follow procedures should have ready access to them. Thus, procedures may be written in job descriptions, employee handbooks, or procedural manuals. Additionally, when procedures are changed or applicable only during a specific time period, they should be properly communicated to those employees responsible for their implementation. By having standardized forms, essential information can also be recorded, processed, and stored more efficiently than when information is communicated by some non-standardized method.
5. To meet environmental changes, procedures must be sufficiently flexible. In fact, managers should constantly review procedures so that .they can be changed as new developments occur. Frequent adjustments in procedures, however, may be sufficient reason to question if they are even needed in the first place.
6. Procedures should reflect alternative courses of action and not be so constrained that flexibility is lost. Options should be made available to incorporate the idea of contingency planning when risks are high.
7. Like policies, good procedures are important coordinating techniques. Coordination, however, depends on procedures that ensure clarity, understanding, adequate records, and internal control.[20]

Many health and fitness managers do not seem to realize the necessity of having well-written procedures. In fact, some managers do have written procedures, but these are not administered adequately. It is important to note that procedures as a planning element are often poorly handled by managers; as a consequence, they demand a great deal more of the manager's attention if goals and objectives are to be realized than if the procedures were properly planned initially.

Rules are regulations or laws that stipulate what personal conduct is required of an employee. They either prescribe or prohibit action by specifying what an employee may or may not do in a given situation.

---

20. Trewatha and Newport, *Management,* pp. 157–158.

Rules are usually accompanied by stated penalties which vary in degree according to the seriousness of the offense and the number of previous violations. Whereas policies serve as the guides in decision making, and procedures prescribe what exact set of actions are to be taken in a particular situation, rules are specific, definite, concrete and leave little or no room for interpretation, judgment, or question. The only element of choice associated with a rule is whether it applies in a given situation. One of the best examples is a rule such as "No Smoking." However, since smoking is usually permitted in designated areas, the rule does not apply to the entire building.[21]

PROGRAM AND PARTICIPATION POLICIES

Authorities in the field of health promotion state emphatically that programs conducted without written policies will eventually run into difficulties. The same fact holds true for people who join a health and fitness program where there are no written policies that apply directly to them. Policies that are clear and easily understood will reduce confusion and misinterpretation and in the long run will make the potential participants feel less apprehensive and more comfortable, particularly if they are registered in a fitness program. On the other hand, policies are not expected to cover every eventuality, as some situations may occur that go beyond the limits of a particular policy statement. When these situations occur, the manager should refer the problem to a higher level of authority.

Because of the differences in size, mission, and types of health and fitness programs, it would be impossible to list all policies that affect the participant and relate to the program. However, the following are some suggested policies, separated into those applicable to both health education and fitness programs and those applicable to fitness programs only:

Policies for Health Education and/or Fitness Programs

- All programs should benefit both the participant and the organization.
- All employees are eligible to participate with approval of immediate supervisor/manager.
- Participation is on employee's own time (or may be on work time depending on the amount of incentive the employer wishes to give).

21. Adapted from Arthur G. Bedeian and William F. Glueck, *Management,* 3rd ed. (New York, NY: The Dryden Press, 1983), pp. 183–184.

- Cost of each program may be paid fully by the organization, the employee, or on a cost-share basis.
- Penalty for not completing a program shall result in the employee paying the full amount if the program is paid fully or partially by the organization.
- Incentives should be given upon completion of a program.
- Participants may register for only one health program and one fitness program at the same time (or some reasonable limit on participation).
- All employees should take part in a health risk appraisal survey or any similar survey.
- All participants' records and data shall be kept confidential.
- Whether or not employees participate in a program will not affect their employment.
- Interest and needs assessments should be done periodically.
- Support group meetings should be an integral part of the program.

Policies for Fitness Programs

In addition to those aforementioned general policies, fitness programs require some unique policies:

- All potential participants must receive medical clearance if they are at high risk or are 40 years or older.
- The potential participant must complete a physical activity profile.
- A complete fitness evaluation—height, weight, muscular strength, muscular endurance, flexibility, pulmonary function, postural strength, and body fat composition—is required of all participants who wish to enter the program.
- A cardiovascular evaluation, either step test, cycle test, or treadmill test, is also required of all participants who wish to enter the program.
- An informed-consent form must be signed by each potential participant entering the program.
- Counseling is an integral part of the program.
- Physician referrals are always welcome.

Policies for Managers

Experts in the field of health and fitness management seem to have overlooked the importance of operating policies for managers and staff in health and fitness programs. Therefore, the following is an attempt to list some suggested operating policies in hopes that they will help managers and their staffs to develop their own. Managers of programs will discover that there can be numerous policies, but they must decide which ones are most appropriate for them in their particular situations.

Personnel Policies

- The manager must know and follow the guidelines developed by the organization when hiring, promoting, or firing full-time or part-time staff, including adhering to all equal employment opportunity and affirmative action requirements.
- The manager must perform an evaluation of each full-time and part-time staff member on a regular basis (at least annually).
- The manager meets with each staff member on a regular basis to review the participants' goals and objectives (at least annually).
- The manager recommends a salary scale for each staff member to his or her supervisor.
- The manager is involved in arbitration, conflicts, or disputes among the staff. If a staff member is in a union, the manager meets with the union representative.
- The manager should develop job descriptions for all positions.
- The manager should promote within the staff when possible.
- The manager should organize in-service training programs.

Fiscal Policies

- The manager develops, submits, and expends the budget (usually approved by his or her superior).
- The manager recommends and/or decides upon purchase of any equipment, supplies, or other materials needed for the program.
- The manager sets fees for programs, if there are fees, but may need to get approval from his or her superior.
- The manager may hire consultants as needed for the program.

Program Management Policies

- The manager schedules all classes and needed space for the program.
- The manager sees that the facilities, if available, are kept clean and maintained.
- The manager provides an admission policy that includes medical clearance for any fitness program.
- The manager must know all the safety procedures associated with the program.
- The manager must know the limits of liability and stay updated to avoid negligence.
- The manager coordinates the program component policies with the comprehensive program policies.
- The manager's policies should be consistent with those of the organization.
- The manager's policies must comply with the goals and objectives of the organization.

Program Promotion Policies

- The manager should represent the program, at various clubs, agencies, or organizations.
- The manager should promote the program through brochures, flyers, or newsletters.

Policies for Staff

In order for any health and fitness program to function efficiently and effectively, it must have a qualified, competent, and satisfied staff. It is the staff member who has the close contact with the participants and is the showcase of the program.

Health and fitness staff personnel must come under the same policies, rules, and procedures as all other employees of the organization. The focus of this section, however, is to list some suggested policies that are applicable to staff personnel associated with a health and fitness program.

- All full-time and part-time fitness staff should know the contents and how to apply the material in the *Y's Way to Physical Fitness* book or, better still, become certified by the American College of Sports Medicine.
- All staff should dress in a professional manner.

- All staff should arrive at least 15 minutes before classes are to begin to set up equipment. After class, they should put back all equipment, supplies or other materials used.
- All instruction should be clear and loud enough for everyone in the class to hear.
- Classes should start and end on time.
- All staff should be qualified, trained, knowledgeable, and skilled at adapting to individual needs.
- All staff must monitor each participant in fitness classes regularly and call for help immediately in case of an emergency.
- All fitness staff must be certified in cardiopulmonary resuscitation.
- All staff must know emergency action procedures and first aid.
- All staff must make the safety of participants their top priority.
- All staff should be covered by liability insurance.
- Staff should not accept gifts or money from any participant or group.

SUMMARY

Standing-use plans include policies, procedures, and rules. Policies are very important in the efficient and effective management of any program or organization. Flexibility, comprehensiveness, coordination, ethical behavior and clarity are the basic characteristics of a clearly defined policy. Procedures are incorporated into policies; yet, policies reflect intent, while procedures show how and when plans are to be carried out. Policies and procedures must be carefully planned before their implementation, and proper communication among the staff and with the manager is essential.

Rules, as well as policies, must be carefully thought out and planned before they are put into effect. They are of vital importance, as they directly affect the conduct of participants. If rules are violated, the employee can expect some kind of penalty, the degree of which depends upon past offenses.

Finally, the chapter concludes by describing more fully some suggested policies which may be helpful for health and fitness managers.

PART III
ORGANIZING THE HEALTH
AND FITNESS PROGRAM

Chapter VI

ORGANIZING THE HEALTH
AND FITNESS PROGRAM: STAFFING

THE ORGANIZING PROCESS

Managers will find that familiarizing themselves with the organizing process, as it relates to a health and fitness program, can be extremely beneficial, since organizing follows planning as another of their responsibilities. A logical beginning is to differentiate between *organization,* the noun, and *organizing,* the verb. An organization may be defined as two or more people working together in a coordinated manner in order to achieve common goals and objectives. Organizing, on the other hand, is a process of bringing together human and physical resources and functions in an orderly, coordinated manner in order to accomplish planned goals and objectives.

As used here, the process of organizing, which should be closely integrated with planning, consists of dividing the required work so as to achieve an effective, efficient, and successful program. Coordination of staff and facilities is imperative if the program is to reach its goals and objectives. When the organizing function is performed effectively, the staff will better understand the goals and objectives of the program, as well as the responsibilities they are to undertake and the functions they are expected to fulfill.

Managers who want to organize a comprehensive health and fitness program should take the following six steps:

• Determine what components are to be offered and set a tentative timetable for each to be implemented. For example, aerobic dance will be offered for ten weeks, starting on October 5.
• Determine who will offer the program and/or how the particular program will be offered and make the assignment if appropriate. For example, the manager assigns a qualified full-time or part-time

87

staff member to teach the smoking-cessation program. If no qualified staff is available, a resource person will need to be hired.

- Decide how to achieve coordination.* Regardless of what components are offered and who teaches them, a need is created to achieve coordination between all personnel and the manager. For example, the instructor of the walk/jog program and the manager must coordinate so as to insure that the facility and equipment are available.
- Decide on a span of control.* The "span of control" of a manager is the number of staff or outside resource personnel who report directly to that person. Deciding on the appropriate span of control is important: Having too few staff or resource personnel may mean the manager's time is not used effectively; too many staff or resource personnel may consume too much of the manager's time.
- Decide how much authority should be delegated.* Managers must make the decision as to how much authority is to be delegated to the staff or resource personnel. For example, a manager may decide that the weight training instructor can select a piece of equipment to be purchased, but it must not cost over $3,000; and the purchase must be approved in advance by the manager.
- Draw an organizational chart.* Once programs to be offered have been finalized and have been assigned, managers should formalize their comprehensive program in an organizational chart. This chart shows the "skeleton" of the entire program in chart form and what programs each staff member or resource person has been assigned. In addition, the manager writes out a job description for each staff member or resource person.[22]

CONSIDERATIONS FOR STAFFING

Rationale for Hiring Staff

Health and fitness programs may be delivered in several different ways; however, organizations would be well advised to hire their own in-house staff, full-time and/or part-time. It has been said many times that no organization can be greater than its employees, nor can a health and fitness program be greater than its staff.

---

*These four steps for organizing a program will be discussed in more detail later in this chapter.

22. Adapted from Gary Dressler, *Management Fundamentals*, 4th ed. (Englewood Cliffs, NJ: Prentice Hall, Inc., 1985), pp. 116–117. Used by permission.

When organizations are considering initiating a comprehensive program, they should also carefully plan what kind of professionals should be hired and the number. Many organizations start with only one or two programs, either health education or fitness, depending on the results of the interest survey and the needs survey and the resources available, and hire either one full-time or one or two part-time staff. It is prudent to begin programming in a small way and add both new or repeat programs and staff personnel as needed.

The hiring of an in-house staff of health and fitness professionals is a step in the right direction for the following major reasons:

- A staff would be more interested, concerned, committed to the program and would realize personal ownership.
- A staff could assist in the planning and organizing programs and in scheduling the health and fitness classes.
- A staff could be formed into a committee or subcommittee to work on special projects or events.
- A staff could become coworkers with the manager and thus provide assistance when necessary.
- A staff could be called together for brainstorming sessions.
- A staff could make communication open and easy.
- A staff would have control of the program and would strive for quality because they have to live with the program.
- A staff would know where the existing resources are and how to utilize them.
- A staff would be more interested in, and concerned with, the participants.
- A staff could be used as role models.
- A staff would cost less in the long run.
- A staff could perform all of the health instruction and lead fitness classes.
- A staff would be more available to answer questions and offer encouragement and could also serve as interviewers and counselors.
- A staff would be aware of equipment and supply needs and could care for the equipment.
- A staff would be more concerned about the facilities, if they are available.
- A staff could conduct the fitness testing and analysis and interpret the results.
- A staff could evaluate each program component.

- A staff could recruit volunteers to lead fitness classes.
- A staff could offer in-service training.
- A staff could provide training to staffs employed at other organizations.

After considering the major reasons for hiring an in-house staff to conduct the health and fitness program, managers would then need to convince top management that this is the best approach. Although other options may be available, the organization which uses its own staff to offer the program will definitely find that it has chosen the best option.

A Functional Health and Fitness Organizational Chart

A functional health and fitness organizational chart is a diagram that depicts the basic arrangement of components within the comprehensive program. The chart also conveys useful information about the program's overall structure by means of a series of connecting lines showing relationships of positions to one another, to the manager, and to the person (department head or employee assistance program head or executive director) to whom the health and fitness manager reports within the organization.

A functional organizational chart should:

- Group jobs together
- Establish formal communication lines
- Show organizational hierarchy (who reports to whom), and
- Name the organizational units.

The above functional organizational chart depicts the basic working relationship between the two units: health education and physical fitness. Its purpose is to show the planned relationships, that is, those thought about and deliberately implemented by the manager and staff after approval by the department head or the employee assistance program head or the executive director. It does not depict informal relationships among the staff, even though these are often at least as significant as the formal relationships.

The organizational structure shown in the chart should be a function of the goals and objectives of the comprehensive program that the manager seeks to achieve and the strategies used to achieve them. In other words, the manager's strategic plan should determine the structure and not vice versa.

Figure 2

Sample Functional Health and Fitness Organizational Chart

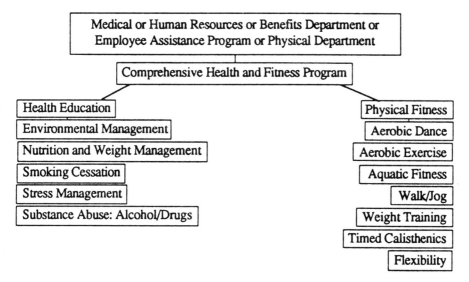

Health and Fitness Staffing Patterns

In any health and fitness staffing pattern, relationships with staff members are extremely significant. The staffing pattern should be flexible; it is effective only if both the staff and the manager are well-motivated and understand and accept their responsibilities within both the program and the organization.

How should a health and fitness staffing pattern be set up? The answer to this question depends upon the organization itself—the size, the extent of top management's commitment to the program, the availability of financial resources and other necessary resources, services available within the organization, and duties required of the staff. All health and fitness programs can function efficiently and effectively under any one of the following three patterns. However, each of the three patterns under which the program is housed depends on the present size of the program and the expansion of the program.

Many organizations have either a medical department, a human resources department, a benefits department, an employee assistance program or a physical department. It is in one of these departments or in the employee assistance program that the health and fitness program may be located and, consequently, to which the manager has reporting responsibilities. Regardless of which level or pattern is utilized, the manager keeps the same reporting responsibilities.

The minimal, or level one, staffing pattern should have the manager reporting to one of the above-mentioned department heads or to the head of the employee assistance program or to the executive director. Usually at this level, one part-time staff member is employed. In addition, a professional advisory committee is selected, hopefully with an in-house physician, if available, as a member of the committee. If an in-house physician is not available, then a medical consultant should be hired to meet periodically with the staff and the manager and should be available by telephone to provide advisement, particularly if fitness programs are being offered. Obviously, if the program is located in the medical department, a physician would already be available to serve on the committee and for consultation.

The second staffing pattern is intermediate, or level two. Here, the manager has the same reporting line as in the minimal structure; but in the intermediate pattern, he or she would employ a staff, whether one full-time or two part-time. At this level there also should be an advisory committee and an in-house physician, if available, as a member of the committee. If an in-house physician is not available, a medical consultant should be hired to meet periodically with the staff and the manager and should be available by telephone to provide advisement, particularly if fitness programs are being conducted.

The third staffing pattern is comprehensive, or level three. In this pattern, the manager has the same reporting responsibilities as in the other two. At this level, he or she would increase the staff to two or more full-time or four or more part-time as needed as the program expands. If the program is not located in the medical department, a medical consultant should be hired to meet periodically with the staff and the manager and should be available by telephone to provide advisement, particularly if fitness programs are being offered. And, of course, the advisory committee is still an important part of the structure.

A health education unit is generally classified as a separate entity within the comprehensive program, yet it functions interdependently with the fitness unit. Health education units utilize the organization's conference room, if available for courses, seminars, and workshops.

A health education unit has two major responsibilities:

Figure 3

Sample of Minimal Health and Fitness
Staffing Patterns Chart

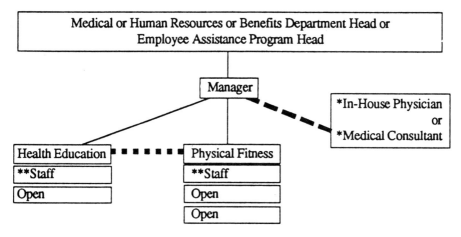

Note: * Serve in an advisory capacity

** One part-time instructional staff depending of the types of programs being offered.

Dashes signify advisement, if fitness programs are being offered.

The dotted line signifies coordination if both health education and fitness programs are being offered.

The boxes marked "open" signify anticipated positions.

1) Planning, developing, and offering a variety of health education courses, seminars, and workshops
2) Coordinating the health education aspects with all of the fitness programs which are being offered.

Fitness programs are usually divided according to physical or health-related components and further divided into fitness rehabilitation components. Cardiovascular endurance or aerobic programs are usually grouped together as are muscular strength and muscular endurance programs. Flexibility exercises may be utilized in both types of programs. These programs, like health education programs, require qualified instructors.

Although a fitness unit may also be classified as a separate entity within the comprehensive program, it still has a close interrelationship with the health education unit. Fitness programs utilize the organization's gymnasium, running track, multi-purpose room, and weight training room, if these are available.

A fitness unit also has two major responsibilities:

1) Planning, developing, and offering several types of fitness programs
2) Coordinating the fitness programs with the health education programs.

Job Analysis

A *job analysis* is the process of identifying the competencies, responsibilities, and experiences needed in the person to fill a position. As a result, it will provide information as to the kind of staff needed. The facts collected about a job form the basis for the development of a job description and a job specification. The analysis is the first step in an effort to identify staff needs; therefore, it should be done carefully and accurately.

Job analysis information can be gathered by several methods that include the following:

- Observation of the job, if not a new position
- Observation of the staff member, if he or she is available
- Examination of previous job analysis and job description, if such are available
- Interview of the staff member, if he or she is available
- Requisition of the staff member to complete an open-ended questionnaire, if he or she is available
- Examination of the log or diary kept by the staff member, if such is available.

The information produced from the job analysis can be used to recruit and select staff personnel, because the manager must know all the specific duties and responsibilities associated with the position. Once managers have performed a job analysis, the task becomes a matter of routine.

Job Descriptions

A fundamental part of the organizing process in any work setting such as a health and fitness program is designing jobs for individual staff members. Once jobs are designed and tasks assigned, it is possible to staff them with human resources, form components, delegate authority, and establish lines of coordination. In many ways, jobs link components together to create the comprehensive program.

A *job* is a collection of tasks performed to support the program's goals and objectives. A *job description* is a written statement which details the duties and responsibilities of the position and includes statement on the following items:

- Duties to be performed
- Supervision given and received
- Relationships with other jobs
- Equipment and materials needed
- Physical working conditions[23]

To be of any value, a job description must be kept up-to-date. It must be complete and, finally, it must include the desired goals and objectives of the job.

Job Specifications

A close partner to the job description is a written document called a *job specification*. The major difference between the two is that job descriptions focus upon the *job,* while the job specification concentrates on the *type of person* required to perform the job.

Usually, the kind of items found in a job specification are the following:

- Education
- Experience
- Oral and written communication
- Initiative
- Judgment
- Physical effort (particularly for fitness staff)
- Personality

---

23. Mondy, Homes, and Flippo, *Management,* p. 276.

When writing a job specification, include only the skills, knowledge and abilities required to perform the job. Inclusion of non-job related personal characteristics opens the door to employee discrimination. Employee discrimination results in expensive legal entanglements and, worse, the systematic avoidance of qualified job applicants. Avoid references to the following in writing job specifications (unless you can clearly demonstrate job-relatedness):

- Gender
- Race
- Religious preference
- National origin and/or ethnic background
- Number of children or plans to have children
- Arrest record
- Height, weight and other physical features
- Relatives working for the firm
- Disabilities (e.g., chronic illnesses such as AIDS)
- Age
- Marital status[24]

Job Specialization

In most situations, managers tend to divide the comprehensive program into health education programs and fitness programs, but for organizational reasons only. When both health education components and fitness components are offered (and in most organizations they are or should be), there is a need to employ staff who have the qualifications and specializations needed to reach the desired goals and objectives. Whether full-time or part-time, the staff or resource personnel must be well qualified in order to offer an effective, comprehensive health and fitness program.

Work Load Analysis

Estimating the types and number of health and fitness components to be offered, the amount of instruction needed, and other responsibilities that are necessary in order that a comprehensive program meet its goals

24. Personal communication with Doctor Richard Grover, Assistant Professor of Business Administration, University of Southern Maine, Portland, Maine, November, 1988.

and objectives is called *work load analysis*. There is no standardized formula for determining work loads for a health and fitness staff. Forecasting the number of staff necessary to instruct and carry out other duties and responsibilities associated with the program is one that managers must confront.

Determining staff work loads can be a sensitive matter. Whenever two or more persons are employed in a health and fitness program, it becomes relatively easy to determine instructional hours; but calculating the work hours involved in interviewing, counseling, and testing (an integral part of all fitness programs) is more complicated. In addition, estimating work hours in planning, developing, and offering seminars and workshops also needs to be translated into a person's work load.

Managers may find in some cases that equalizing and giving hour values to work loads is difficult, as frequently assigned tasks may not be given hour values. Health and fitness positions with respect to work loads need more study. At the present time, the best that managers can do is to be fair in making judgments of the work required of staff member(s) or resource personnel. Work loads in health and fitness are not like those in business and industry where work loads are usually quite well established. In some cases, conflicts may arise between one or more of the staff. Difficult situations must be resolved by managers, and attempts should be made to keep these individuals content so that they enjoy their work and feel that they are an important part of a team.

Coordination

Coordination is the process of linking together staff activities toward the accomplishment of the goals and objectives of the comprehensive health and fitness program. It involves making an efficient, effective, and smooth-working team of all health and fitness personnel. Coordination provides for proper communication among all personnel and programs. If the comprehensive program has several components within it, each program may then be assigned a coordinator. It is important to note, however, that coordinators are usually more effective when they possess a variety of skills that can be used to bring about coordination and resolution of conflict.

Both horizontal and vertical coordination is required in the program if coordinators have been assigned. *Vertical coordination* refers to the development of effective integrated relationships between program coordinators and the manager. *Horizontal coordination* is the development of smooth relationships between program coordinators.[25] If staff personnel have been assigned coordinating roles within certain programs, and if they coordinate between programs (horizontal) and report to the manager (vertical) who in turn reports to his or her supervisor within the organization, this type of structure is called *matrix.* Other names given to reporting in a comprehensive program are *chain of command* or *hierarchy of authority.*

How can coordination best be improved? The following procedures may aid the manager:

• Coordination by organizational charts and statements of job descriptions: Health and fitness staff members must know to whom they report, what their jobs are, and what their relationships to other members are. Moreover, they must have a clear understanding of exactly what each other staff member does, particularly if that person is involved in two or more programs.

• Coordination by goals and objectives: Most managers will assist their staff members in establishing goals and objectives to facilitate coordination. When staff members achieve their goals and objectives, their efforts are coordinated because their achievements are reflected in programs which attract an increasing number of participants.

• Coordination by rules or procedures: If managers plan in advance the work that needs to be done, the responsibility of each health and fitness staff person can be specified. Thus, rules and procedures are useful for coordinating routine and recurring activities. They spell out in detail exactly what each staff member must do if a particular situation should arise.

• Coordination by chain of command: In addition to utilizing rules, procedures, goals, and objectives, many health and fitness managers use the chain of command to achieve coordination. Then when situations arise that are not covered, staff personnel are instructed to take the problem to the manager. Utilizing the chain of command to achieve coordination when the manager needs to make a decision works well as long as the number of problems brought to his or her attention is kept to a minimum.

• Coordination by adequate communication: It is imperative that there be good communication between the health and fitness staff and

25. Adapted from Henry L. Tosi and Stephen J. Carroll, *Management,* 2nd ed. (New York, NY: John Wiley and Sons, 1982), p. 482.

the manager. Changes in plans, procedures, rules, policies, and schedules must become known to all personnel. In cases of emergencies and temporary changes, the manager is responsible and must see that all staff members receive the information immediately.

Regular staff meetings provide a mechanism for disseminating information. Minutes of each staff meeting should be written up and distributed to all staff. Thus, full-time and part-time staff members who were not able to attend the meeting will know exactly what transpired.

Sometimes, a committee or a task force is formed for special projects such as a conference or workshop. Minutes of these meetings should also be written up and made available to all personnel. If the comprehensive health and fitness program is large, all written communication such as memoranda, newsletters, and special reports should be distributed to all staff members. A bulletin board that is available to all staff personnel and looked at frequently is helpful in any written communication effort. One must not overlook the fact that oral communication can also be effective.

• Coordination by proper management: Managers must know what is going on in each component of the comprehensive program and where the problems are in coordination. It is when managers are unaware of what is happening within the program that difficulties in coordination appear. Thus, it becomes necessary that managers keep in fairly close contact with the health and fitness staff in order to develop good relationships, resolve any problems, and correct any misunderstandings before these create a poor working environment.

• Coordination by voluntary interaction: Coordination is always enhanced when all health and fitness staff members are working toward the betterment of the program. Proper attitude and high morale will make coordination smooth. Pride in the program and in the organization will usually make personnel relinquish their self-interests and thereby help coordination.

Voluntary interaction is developed when staff members get to know and understand one another. When personnel accept the working ways and speaking customs of others, they improve working relationships.

Informal contacts, such as breaks, lunch, health education classes, exercise sessions, and locker room conversations, provide excellent opportunities to supplement formal communication. Friendly and social relationships between staff members not only promote voluntary adjustments but also aid in achieving better coordination.

Span of Control

The number of staff who report to the manager is referred to as the *span of control*. With wide spans, the manager has a relatively large number of personnel who report directly. In contrast, in narrow spans, there are relatively few who report directly. Wide spans are challenging to the manager as they broaden the program, but narrow spans tend to expedite more interpersonal staff-manager relationships.[26]

How many staff can a manager of a health and fitness program effectively supervise? Stated in different words: What is the proper span of control necessary to oversee a comprehensive health and fitness program? There are no definitive answers to these questions. A specific number of staff reporting to a manager cannot be determined because of the following factors:

• The competence of both the manager and the staff: The more competent they are, the wider the span of control.

• The degree of interaction that is required between and among the programs to be supervised: The more required interaction, the narrower the span of control must be.

• The extent to which the manager must carry out non-managerial tasks: The more instructing the manager has to do, the less time is available for supervising others. Thus, the span of control must be narrow.

• The relative similarity or dissimilarity of the jobs being supervised: The more similar the jobs or programs, the wider the span of control can be; the more dissimilar the jobs or programs, the narrower the span of control must be.

• The extent of standardized procedures: The more routine or standardized instructional procedures of the staff are, and the greater the degree to which each job is performed by standardized methods, the wider the span of control can be.

• The degree of physical dispersion: If all the staff are located in one area, the manager can supervise more staff than if the staff is dispersed throughout a fitness facility and in a conference room.[27]

---

26. Adapted from Terry and Franklin, *Principles of Management.* p. 207.

27. Ivancevich, Donnelly, and Gibson, *Management for Performance,* pp. 180–181.

Delegation of Authority

In cases where managers are overloaded with work and additional help is required, how is this type of situation handled? The answer is simply to delegate authority in three different ways: First, select a staff member and assign him or her some of the managerial duties. Second, if several components are being offered, name a coordinator from the staff to each; and lastly, if funds are available, hire an assistant manager. When authority is delegated, the issue becomes the choice of an individual or individuals who can make decisions, at times without approval of the manager.

The question arises as to whether or not a health and fitness program should be centralized or decentralized. It is strongly recommended that the comprehensive program be centralized with one budget and a manager reporting to an appropriate department head or head of the employee assistance program. If the program becomes large enough, an assistant manager may be hired and some duties and responsibilities may be delegated to that person. However, the assistant manager should not make decisions without first attaining the approval of the manager. In such cases where large programs are being conducted and coordinators are designated, the coordinators report to the assistant. When and if authority is delegated, it must be clearly understood what power, if any, that individual has to make decisions without first consulting the manager.

Forecasting Staff Requirements

Forecasting is a process in which managers calculate and predict future staff needs. Staffing is one of the responsibilities of a health and fitness manager and requires hiring qualified instructors or resource personnel to work in the program. However, forecasting can also be utilized in other aspects of the program in addition to staffing, for example, office space allocation, facilities, equipment, and supplies. All types of forecasting must be predicated on future needs, and in some cases what was forecasted as being needed may not be actually needed at all. However, the responsibility for forecasting is one that all managers should not neglect.

Staff planning and forecasting requires consideration of a variety of internal as well as external factors. Rate of program growth, personnel turnover, budget, scope of health and fitness programs are critical internal factors to consider. Demographic characteristics of the relevant labor market, availability of qualified applicants, level of competition for labor, and level of client demand for services are external factors that must be carefully identified and evaluated.[28]

Recruitment

Whether starting a health and fitness program or filling a position in an existing program, the manager is basically responsible for recruitment of personnel. *Recruitment,* as used here, is a process that involves searching for qualified staff to fill either a health education or a fitness position or both. But before any search begins, a word of caution: Managers must adhere to the equal employment opportunity and the affirmative action requirements.

The process of recruitment involves the following:

- Whenever possible, promote from within the program if a candidate is qualified. This process is popular with the staff and serves as an incentive for possible advancement. Steps for advancement should be established early.
- Advertise in the local newspapers and professional journals to reach those who would not otherwise know of the opening.
- Recruit at colleges and universities that grant degrees in either health science or exercise science or both. The applicants received from these sources should have satisfactory backgrounds and they should improve as they gain more experience.
- Recruit from other organizations that have health and fitness programs. Health and fitness professionals are mobile and seek advancement.
- A staff member or a participant may refer someone who is qualified for the position(s). Be aware that participants are not always good judges of the qualifications of the applicants.
- Walk-ins may apply for the position(s).

The advantages of promoting from within the program are:

- The price of recruiting is lower.
- The staff member is already familiar with the program.
- The staff member's performance record is already established.
- Incentive and motivation are present.
- Loyalty is strengthened.

---

28. Grover, personal communication.

On the other hand, there are disadvantages such as:

- Fewer new ideas
- Jealousy among staff, and
- Possible stagnation.

The advantages of hiring outside the program are:

- Fresh ideas
- New approaches, and
- Diversity.

On the other hand, there are disadvantages such as:

- Recruiting can be costly.
- Outside hiring may upset present staff members.
- Checking previous work record is time consuming.
- Orientation and training can be costly.[29]

Selection

Selection is a process that involves a series of steps beginning with screening and ending with managers hiring personnel to fill either a new position(s) or an existing vacancy. The selection of health and fitness personnel depends to a great extent upon programmatic needs and, again, must comply with both state and federal legal requirements.

The steps in the selection process include the following:

- Application forms. These forms are useful for gathering information and historical data about candidates. The form contains such items as personal data, education, prior experience and references. The application form is generally reviewed by the human resources department and, in some cases, by the manager to determine whether the person is generally qualified for the position.
- Resumes. A screening tool which has become popular in recent years is the resume. It is a good device for reviewing the candidate's background, education, and experience. Resumes are usually much more comprehensive than the application form.
- Committees. Some managers like the idea of getting assistance from committees for screening application forms or resumes. Committees are now used extensively and are highly recommended. Some man-

---

29. Adapted from Terry and Franklin, *Principles of Management*, pp. 273–275.

agers prefer having two screening committees, namely, initial and final; while others feel one committee, a final, does suffice.

When managers of health and fitness programs choose to have two screening committees, the initial is usually composed of a staff member, if available, a nurse, and several other employees, one from each department, who are interested in the program. This committee's responsibility is to screen out the applications and/or resumes and select the top five or six applicants they judge to have the best qualifications. These names are then forwarded on to the final committee. This committee decides whether or not they wish to design a written rating scale. The final screening committee is usually composed of a staff member, if available, a nurse or physician, if available, and a representative from the human resources department.

It is strongly recommended that this committee design a written scale to rate the candidates. The scale is an effort to be more objective rather than depend totally on subjective, off-the-cuff judgments. It is important that the rating scale be simple, clear, and concise and that the committee have a good understanding of the criteria and screening process. The criteria for selection is based on the job description and job specification. The major responsibility of this committee is to agree as to who the three or four most qualified applicants are.

- Managers. Because in the final analysis health and fitness managers must decide from the applications or resumes which candidate is the most qualified, some prefer to eliminate the committee(s) in the selection process. They feel that committee(s) are too time consuming and the task of getting employees to serve becomes a major problem. Many employees do not like to serve on committees, particularly on their own time. As a result, some managers prefer to do their own screening of applicants to select the most qualified candidate.

While managers are going through the screening of applicants, they should be in constant communication with their supervisors. It should be noted that in small organizations with small programs, managerial screening and selecting of staff may work out well. However, in large organizations with large programs, the committee(s) selection process is advisory, with managers making the final decision.

- Interviews. Personal interviews are an integral part of any selection process and considered the most important step. The interview can elicit more types of information, such as communication skills, physical appearance, and mannerisms, than it is possible to gather from application forms or resumes. The interviewing of applicants may be accomplished in two different ways: First, the manager may wish to have the final screening committee members participate in all the interviews and use their judgment as a basis for selection. Secondly, health and fitness managers may wish to conduct all the interviews in order to make a final decision.

  After the first round of interviews and the choice is narrowed down to two or three, a second interview of these final candidates may take place. The second interviews must be carried out exactly like the first, i.e., either by the final screening committee or by the manager. The second interviews may focus on such topics as the philosophy of health and fitness, participants' attitudes, changing life-styles, staffing and facilities.

  Basically, there are three types of interviews: *structured*, in which specific questions are predetermined; *semistructured*, in which only some questions are predetermined; and *unstructured*, in which there are no set questions or topics that are predetermined. It is important that all applicants in the structured and semistructured interviews be asked the same set of questions. Both the semistructured and unstructured interviews allow for flexibility, as they give applicants an opportunity to ask questions rather than just answer questions.

- Hiring Decision. The final step in the selection process is the decision to hire. After all the candidates have been interviewed and assessed, references, if any, checked, and letters of recommendation reviewed, managers are now ready to make the final decision as to who will be hired. Managers should first recommend the candidate to their department head or to the employee assistance program head. If approved, the name of the candidate selected is forwarded to the human resources department, which does the processing. The person who is hired should then be introduced to the staff and to any other personnel with whom he or she will be associated.

Promotions

Some of the long-range decisions managers must concern themselves with are promotions, as promotions impact upon the professional growth of the individual staff member and on the program. A *promotion,* as used here, means a move up in the organizational structure of the program wherein the person is usually given greater responsibility and an increase in salary. In addition, a staff member usually finds that a promotion helps satisfy the need for achievement, challenge, and self-esteem. "Ideally, one would like to see a promotion program that is fair, free from bias and discrimination."[30]

In some programs, managers promote a staff member on merit and/or seniority. However, most managers of health and fitness programs prefer to base staff promotions on performance evaluations. Regardless of which basis for promotion is used, managers must take into consideration union guidelines, if present, and also the organization's guidelines.

Figure 4

Sample Comprehensive Health and Fitness Program
Staff Promotional Chart

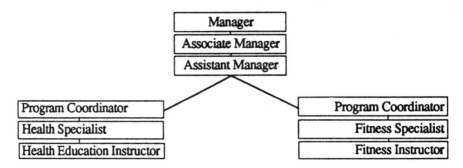

In-House Physician or Medical Consultant

If organizations are conducting various types of fitness programs, it then is crucial that they have an in-house physician or they must hire a medical consultant. Since large organizations usually employ one or more full-time physicians, top management can very well talk over with

---

30. Andrew D. Szilagyi, Jr., *Management and Performance.* 2nd ed. (Glenview, IL: Scott, Foresman and Co., 1984), p. 558.

them their responsibilities associated with the fitness programs so as to provide medical consultation. Experience has shown that in contemporary times trying to recruit volunteers as medical consultants to fitness programs is almost impossible.

Fitness programs should never be designed and implemented without the assistance of medical consultants. Furthermore, it is important that whoever does the medical consulting should possess the following characteristics:

- Have a strong commitment to the organization's fitness programs
- Have strong convictions that the organization's fitness programs are beneficial and are an integral part of the participant's holistic health
- Must be actively practicing medicine in the community, if a hired medical consultant
- Should possess the ability to communicate essential medical information to the staff and manager
- Should be enthusiastic when speaking to employees about the value of exercise
- Should serve as a member of the advising committee, if in-house physician

The duties of an in-house physician or medical consultant are as follows:

- Assists in designing fitness programs
- Assists with the development of all medical policies and procedures for the fitness programs
- Is available to answer medical questions by phone and give advice
- Assists with the emergency action procedures
- Gives, in some cases, medical approval on certain participants
- Meets with the staff and manager if necessary to discuss participants who have medical problems.

As previously mentioned, whether there are in-house physicians or hired medical consultants, managers should never start any type of fitness program without medical advisement. There are inherent, in fitness programs, participants who should be closely monitored because of medical problems.

Volunteers

When there is a shortage of instructors for fitness programs, the staff or perhaps the manager may train some of the participants and/or student interns to be class leaders. These class leaders are not actually replacement for the staff, but volunteers who are trained as class leaders can be of tremendous value since they can give staff members time to perform other duties such as testing, interviewing, and counseling. However, the recruitment of volunteers and their training are time consuming.

What would a staff member look for in volunteers? The potential volunteer class leaders should possess the following characteristics:

- They should have a strong belief in the value and benefits derived from exercise.
- They should be regular participants in fitness programs, attending three times a week.
- They should be in good physical condition and seen as models.
- They should be cognizant of the various needs and limitations of participants.
- They should be energetic and pleasant.
- They should help participants learn how to appreciate physical activity.
- They should be capable of helping participants realize the social benefits that can be derived from attending fitness classes.[31]

SUMMARY

The organizing process, which is closely integrated with planning, provides managers with some valuable information. Six steps for organizing a comprehensive health and fitness program are necessary.

Organizations would be well advised to hire their own staff to conduct the health and fitness program. This chapter introduces many important reasons for employing an in-house staff as opposed to other alternatives.

A functional health and fitness organizational chart is a diagram that provides information about the comprehensive program's overall structure by a series of connecting lines. These lines show relationships of positions to one another, to the manager, and to the person to whom the manager reports.

---

31. Adapted from Lawrence A. Golding, Clayton R. Myers and Wayne E. Sinning, *The Y's Way to Physical Fitness*, Revised (Chicago, IL: National Board of YMCA, 1982), p. 36.

Health and fitness staffing patterns are discussed. They are divided into three levels. In all levels, the manager of a health and fitness program reports to an appropriate department head or to the head of the employee assistance program. The number of staff usually determines the level.

A sample of a comprehensive health and fitness program staff promotion chart is illustrated. Also included in this chart are titles and promotional steps.

The chapter ends by discussing a variety of topics that health and fitness managers should consider when they are addressing the issue of staffing. Also, the topic of volunteers and their role with respect to fitness programs is taken up.

Chapter VII

ORGANIZING THE HEALTH AND FITNESS PROGRAM: FACILITIES AND EQUIPMENT

INTRODUCTION

The extent to which organizations are committed to a health and fitness program, both philosophically and financially, will dictate the type(s) of facilities and the amount of equipment needed. Health and fitness facilities and equipment can range from a small conference or meeting room equipped only with an overhead projector for conducting health education programs to a medium-sized gymnasium with an adjacent weight training room, men's and women's showers, toilets, drying areas, lockers, women's makeup room, and offices. With respect to equipment, a weight training machine, two rowing ergometers, a treadmill, and at least two computerized stationary bicycles for conducting fitness programs are recommended.

Because organizations vary as to size, number of employees, type of employees, financial resources, and the newness of health and fitness programs, it would be unrealistic even to attempt to set standards for facilities and equipment. Moreover, some organizations have both fitness and recreation programs, a fact which makes the task of setting standards for health and fitness facilities and equipment almost impossible. Therefore, in most cases, it can be said that from organization to organization there will be a great deal of variation pertaining to the facilities and the amount and types of equipment required.

Organizations would be well advised that, where circumstances make it feasible, the ideal for promoting health and fitness is through on-site facilities and equipment ownership. However, it is not necessary

---

Note: Because at the present time there are no set standards for renovating existing space or planning for new facilities specifically for fitness programs, the following book is recommended: *Planning Facilities for Athletics, Physical Education and Recreation*, Revised 1985, Richard B. Flynn, Editor and Contributing Author, The Athletic Institute, 200 Castlewood Drive, North Palm Beach, FL 33408 and American Alliance for Health, Physical Education, Recreation and Dance, 1900 Association Drive, Reston, VA 22091.

that both be in place at one time; they may be phased in over a 3–5 year period. On-site facilities are preferred for five important reasons:

- They clearly demonstrate that the organization is interested, concerned, and cares for the health and physical well-being of its employees by funding a facility.
- The convenience of having on-site facilities may interest more employees to participate.
- Scheduling of program(s) may be designed to accommodate any work shifts.
- Existing custodial personnel are available to maintain the attractiveness of the facility.
- They provide an opportunity for the spouses and families of employees to participate in the program(s).

To assist managers in estimating space, excluding swimming pools, the following guidelines should be considered:

- Estimate the number of participants who will be utilizing the space on both a per-class daily basis and also on a weekly basis.
- If a room, estimate the amount of space that is necessary for a single participant to perform a particular exercise or activity.
- If a complete gymnasium complex, determine floor markings according to the recreational, intramural and interorganizational sports programs that may be offered.
- If a complete gymnasium complex, provide a storage area conveniently located for security of equipment—bicycle ergometers, rowing ergometers, mats, and so forth.
- Locate showers, drying areas, lockers, lavatories, storage room, toilets, and women's makeup room close to the main floor so that they are easily accessible.
- If a room, estimate the circulation space so as to allow participants to come in and leave the area without disturbing other participants.
- Determine what sound control and acoustics are required.
- Determine whether hardwood or synthetic floor surface is more suitable for the programs and activities that are to be offered. New synthetic surfaces are becoming very popular for floors subject to heavy usage.
- Determine ceiling heights by the exercise or activity requirements.
- If a room, estimate the amount of space needed for the instructor.

As has been mentioned previously in another chapter, managers of health and fitness programs have several responsibilities, among which are finding available space, organizing a facility, and purchasing equipment. Obviously, in order for a health and fitness program to be successful, facilities and equipment are absolute necessities. Predicated upon the philosophy that organizations should have on-site facilities, whenever possible, and equipment ownership, whenever possible, managers need to consider the following seven important questions and recommended responses:

1. What facilities and equipment are needed? Analyzing the results of the interest survey and needs survey will determine the facilities and equipment needed. Managers can then ascertain not only what programs should be offered but also, just as important, what facilities and equipment are needed.

2. How are facilities and equipment acquired? Managers of health and fitness programs must "sell," or convince, top management that total funding for a facility and equipment is crucial and can make the difference as to whether or not the program is successful. Another approach is to request total funding in advance from top management. Then the organization can partially or fully repay the money by imposing a fee for each program(s) employees wish to enter. Of course, repaying the organization is a long-term project. Some managers have generated additional financial resources by sponsoring various types of special events. These additional resources could be used in several different ways in an effort to help support a comprehensive health and fitness program. A listing of these special events is mentioned in Chapter IX. However, managers would be well advised to convince top management, if possible, to provide total funding for a facility, equipment, and supplies.

3. What rooms or areas should be included in a facility? The amount of funding and the number and kinds of employees will determine the rooms or areas to be included. A complete gymnasium complex, including, in addition to the main floor, a conference or classroom, a weight training room, an aerobic exercise room, men's and women's locker rooms, showers, drying areas, toilets, a women's makeup room, and a storage room, would be most ideal. The gymnasium could also be used for open recreation, intramural sports, interorganizational sports, dances, and as an auditorium. If there is only a medium or large size room, then adjacent to this room should be locker rooms, a women's makeup room, showers, drying areas, and toilets.

4. What are the priorities for selecting facilities? The programs to be offered, funding, and the number and kinds of employees will decide the priorities for selecting facilities. The first priority would be a gymnasium complex; second would be a weight training room; third would be an aerobic exercise room; and fourth would be a swimming pool.

5. What on-site space is available? Managers must conduct a thorough search within the organization's building(s) for any space that could be used for offering health and fitness programs. A few examples are a conference or meeting room, storage room, or an area in the basement.

6. How will the on-site facility help to meet the goals and objectives of the program? An on-site facility will be more convenient, more easily scheduled, and more accessible.

7. What is the alternative if there are no on-site facilities? Lacking an on-site facility, an organization could rent community-based facilities and use its own staff. Secondly, the organization could subsidize fully, or in part, the fee for employees who participate in various programs at a community-based facility and not use its own staff. Employees thus subsidized must complete the program.

It is evident that many managers are seeking information on health and fitness facilities and equipment because of the newness of these types of programs. Therefore, the following sections in this chapter will present general descriptions of health education facilities and both indoor and outdoor fitness facilities. A general description of swimming pools and a checklist for swimming pools will follow. In addition, both health education equipment and fitness equipment, with their purposes, will be listed. The last section will offer a brief discussion of community-based facilities as an alternative to on-site facilities.

FACILITIES FOR HEALTH EDUCATION PROGRAMS

Utilizing the Existing Conference or Meeting Room

When it comes to utilizing a room for offering health education programs, new construction is usually not necessary. As a matter of fact, most organizations already have a conference or meeting room that could be used for delivering health education instruction. Although the room's primary purpose is to hold seminars, meetings, consultations, and discussions, prudent managers, while organizing programs, should investigate scheduling the organization's conference or meeting room for delivering health education programs.

Conference or meeting rooms may be either rectangular, square, or round, and they come in a variety of sizes. Architects suggest fifteen square feet per person to be used as a yardstick. Regardless of the shape, basically there are two types of seating arrangements: The first is the type which allows participants to sit on regular chairs or table armchairs facing the front of the room, as in a conventional school classroom. This type will be most ideal for offering health education programs.

The second type has a table located in the middle of the room around which participants sit facing one another. Although not preferred, this type can be used. A conference or meeting room may not be ideal for offering health education programs; but in many situations, with some modifications, it can suffice.

HEALTH EDUCATION EQUIPMENT

The following is a list of health education equipment and the purposes for which such equipment may be utilized for health education programs:

- Anatomical charts—both male and female, used to show the parts of the human body
- Easel pads—used for writing
- Opaque projector—projects images from books, pictures, loose-leaf flyers onto a screen
- Overhead projector—projects images from transparencies onto a screen
- Plastic human organs and body parts—used to give a more realistic picture of organs and body parts (three-dimensional)
- Screen—used to project pictures upon
- 16mm projector—projects 16mm movies onto a screen (includes audio)
- Slide projector—projects 35mm slides onto a screen
- Videocassette recorder, camera, and monitor—records and/or plays back audio and visual images. In recording, the camera and microphones are needed; when playing back, the videocassette deck. The

deck must be connected to a monitor onto which the images are projected.

INDOOR FACILITIES FOR FITNESS

Facilities play an extremely important role when fitness programs are to be offered. When such fitness facilities are available, they tend to impact favorably upon participants who are already enrolled in health education programs. As a resultant, more employees tend to enter fitness programs.

Regardless of geographic location and climatic conditions, experts in the fitness field agree that facilities are essential if these programs are to be successful. Without fitness facilities, a comprehensive health and fitness program cannot reach its goals and objectives.

The cost of a fitness facility is approximately 30–50 percent of the total cost of a comprehensive program, depending on whether existing space is utilized or new construction is required. Of course, the key to realizing a fitness facility depends to a large extent on the manager. It is he or she who must prepare a strong and well-written proposal to be presented to top management indicating that a fitness facility is vital to the offering of fitness programs.

Utilizing an Existing On-Site Area

It has been said many times that when managers are looking for a space in which to conduct fitness programs, they first should start by exploring on-site areas. Often, they seem inadvertently to overlook the possibility of an on-site space that could be utilized. Depending on the design(s) of the organization's building(s), there may be a storage room, a staff lounge, or an area in the basement available. Depending on their primary usage, these areas could be used on either a full-time or part-time basis. Showers and locker rooms already available would give fitness programs a big boost. Managers should be cognizant of the fact that existing on-site areas usually need some modifications. Any existing on-site areas should be examined closely before any decision is made with respect to implementing any of the fitness programs.

Many organizations have cafeterias. Whenever circumstances permit and conditions are appropriate, these can be used to conduct cardiovascular endurance or aerobic fitness programs at select hours. All that needs to be done is to move the tables and chairs in preparation for each class session. A word of caution about floors of cafeterias: If the composition of the floor is a hard surface, participants may get shin splints.

Some organizations have a recreation room which may be suitable for conducting fitness programs. Depending upon the number and type(s) of recreation equipment housed there, the room could very well be appropriate for selected types of aerobic fitness programs. Obviously, since recreation rooms will vary in size, managers of health and fitness programs should examine the room closely before scheduling any classes.

If there is no existing on-site area for conducting fitness programs, two options are open: The first is to construct a new facility, and the second is to use community-based facilities. The next three topics will deal with new facilities.

A Complete Gymnasium Complex

The facility that can accommodate most of the fitness programs, with the exception of an aquatic fitness program, is a complete gymnasium complex. As to the size of the building, the recommended responses to the first and third questions indicated in the introduction of this chapter may provide the managers with information as to what the dimensions of a gymnasium complex should be. Managers may also use the following floor dimensions:

Bucher suggests for junior and senior high school gymnasiums that floor sizes may vary from a minimum floor space of 48 × 66 feet with one teaching station to a maximum floor space of 66 × 96 feet with two teaching stations, exclusive of the bleachers.[32] These dimensions can be used for small- to medium-sized gymnasium floors.

For colleges and universities, floor sizes are based on total undergraduate enrollment and space requirements are 8.5 to 9.5 square feet per student. A minimum of a 22-foot high ceiling is recommended.[33] These dimensions are suitable for larger gymnasium floors.

Irrespective of floor size, adjacent to the main gymnasium floor should be a weight training room, men's and women's locker and shower rooms,

---

32. Charles A. Bucher, *Administration of Physical Education and Athletic Programs,* 8th ed. (St. Louis, MO: The C.V. Mosby Co., 1983), p. 404.

33. Richard B. Flynn, Editor and Contributing Author. *Planning Facilities for Athletics, Physical Education, and Recreation,* Rev. 1985 (North Palm Beach, FL: The Athletic Institute and Reston, VA: American Alliance for Health, Physical Education, Recreation and Dance), pp. 41–42.

drying areas, a women's makeup room, toilets, an equipment storage room, and an office(s) based on the estimated number of staff anticipated.

In addition to utilizing a gymnasium for fitness programs, the facility can also be used for recreational purposes. Some activities that could be conducted in the facility, depending on the floor markings, are badminton, basketball, tennis, and volleyball. Ballroom, folk, and square dancing are also activities that can be offered.

Weight Training Room

If managers proceed with the organizing of indoor fitness facilities and come to the realization that a complete gymnasium complex is absolutely impossible, the next priority should be a weight training room. The rationale for a weight training room as the second priority is its versatility. That is to say, this room can be used not only for the development of muscular strength and muscular endurance but also for the development of cardiovascular endurance or aerobic conditioning when the appropriate equipment is available. Physical fitness tests may also be administered in a weight training room if the needed testing equipment is on hand.

"A minimum size of 24 feet by 40 feet has been suggested for an exercise room by the President's Council on Physical Fitness and Sports (PCPFS)."[34] This size room would be appropriate as a weight training room.

It is important in organizing a weight training room to give considerable attention to the placement of equipment once the size of the room has been decided. Space in this room should be allocated so that the participants can stretch or warm up prior to using the weight training equipment. Obviously, the number, type, and size of each piece of equipment must coincide with the dimensions of the weight training room. Moreover, enough space needs to be allocated so that participants are not bumping one another while exercising. The floor surface of a weight training room may be either hardwood or synthetic. However, in contemporary times, synthetic floors are becoming popular. It is recommended that 3/4-inch plywood be placed under all machines. If free weights are going to be used, 3/4-inch plywood should also be placed

---

34. "Where to Begin: A Basic Guide to Planning An Employee Fitness Program," *Athletic Purchasing and Facilities*, 4:7, 30, July, 1980.

under the squat racks and platforms, including storage racks. This use of plywood disperses the weight of the weight training equipment over a larger area so as to prevent damage to the floor. The ¾-inch plywood under the squat racks and platforms should be covered with ½-inch hard rubber to prevent damage to the plywood.

Aerobic Exercise Room

The major reason for an aerobic exercise room being the third priority is its relatively limited use. It is obvious that its only use is for aerobic dance, aerobic exercise, regular calisthenics, timed calisthenics, and flexibility programs. Because of financial constraints, top management of some organizations have made the decision that an aerobic exercise room will suffice for selected fitness program offerings. Fitness equipment and maintenance are both quite expensive, whereas the equipment needed for an aerobic exercise room is an AM/FM/radio/stereo cassette recorder.

Aerobic exercise rooms, like weight training rooms, vary in size. George Pfeiffer, former program manager, Xerox Health Management Program, believes that an aerobic area should allow at least 16 square feet per person.[35]

During the last five years, several studies have been undertaken on aerobic floor surfaces. Basically, there are two kinds of aerobics: low-impact and high-impact. Injuries received from both these kinds of aerobics have caused concern and initiated studies on aerobic floor surfaces. In addition, the proper shoes for aerobics are receiving much attention. Doctor Richie, a podiatrist who has written extensively on aerobics and fitness-related topics, reveals the following:

> In programs integrating low-impact aerobics, the surface friction properties of the floor become more important while the shock-absorbing qualities become inconsequential. Highly cushioned, padded-carpet systems designed to dissipate vertical impact stress are least desirable for low-impact aerobics in which lateral movements dominate. A smooth, even, non-yielding surface provides uninhibited foot glide and a stable base of support. For this reason, finished hardwood floors are preferable for programs offering only low-impact aerobics. Floating, padded

---

35. Ruth Halcomb, "Fitness By Design," Reprinted from *Corporate Fitness and Recreation*, 3:4, 18, June/July, 1984, with the permission of Brentwood Publishing Corp., a Prentice-Hall/Simon and Schuster unit of Gulf & Western, Inc.

or spring hardwood floors are recommended for programs which combine low- and high-impact aerobics.[36]

Swimming Pools

Upon investigating organizations that are planning to construct swimming pools, it is evident that managers of health and fitness programs are relied upon to provide top management with at least general information on pool construction and its operation. Aquatic fitness programs are a vital part of a comprehensive health and fitness program. Moreover, swimming can provide an exercise program for those employees who, because of various physical reasons, cannot participate in weight-bearing fitness programs. Furthermore, aquatic fitness programs are preferred by many employees who do not have medical limitations. In addition to the aquatic fitness programs, a swimming pool will provide employees with fun and enjoyment during recreational swim periods.

When writing on the topic of indoor swimming pools, Bucher points out the following:

> Major design decisions must be made if an organization decides to construct a pool. These include such items as the nature of the program to be conducted in a pool type of overflow system, dimension and shape of pool, depth of the water, type of finish, type of filters and water treatment system, construction material, amount of deck area, climate control, illumination, and number of spectators to be accommodated.[37]

As health and fitness managers read the above, it becomes evident that the last major design decision, the number of spectators, may or may not be applicable for organizations planning to construct a swimming pool. Obviously, there is no need for a spectator gallery if only aquatic fitness programs and recreation swim periods are offered. Organizations that include families in their health and fitness programs should invite them to use the pool during the hours it is not being used by employees. Again, a spectator gallery is not necessary. If, on the other hand, organizations decide to rent their swimming facilities for competitive swimming, it is absolutely necessary that a spectator gallery be included in the construction plans.

---

36. Douglas H. Richie, Jr., "Aerobic Floor Surfaces." Reprinted from *Corporate Fitness and Recreation*, 5, 5:55, Aug./Sept., 1986, with permission of Brentwood Publishing Corp., a Prentice-Hall/Simon and Schuster unit of Gulf & Western, Inc.

37. Bucher, *Physical Education Programs*, p. 406.

At this point, the following discussion will focus on the general guiding principles of pool construction and operation. It is important that managers keep in mind the instructional and recreational needs of employees who register for the aquatics fitness programs.

Piscopo, a former swimmer, swimming coach, and presently a swimming meet official and an author, has put forth some valuable information relative to swimming pools:

> In most climates, an indoor pool is preferred; otherwise, instruction and recreational swimming must be curtailed during the winter months. The size of pools vary from 30 × 60 feet to 60 × 75 feet. Some pools are Olympic size (50 meters long). Unfortunately, too many pools are 30 feet wide with four lanes, which severely restrict the number of swimmers who can use the facility at one time.
>
> Pools that contain six to eight lane widths and 75 foot lengths are more functional from an instructional perspective, and should be supported in the planning and construction stages. Safe water depths range from two feet six inches to four and one-half feet at the shallow end; and from ten to twelve feet at the deep end. Standard water depths of three feet six inches (shallow end) and twelve feet (deep end) are recommended to meet the instructional and recreational needs of most swimmers.
>
> Pools equipped with a one meter diving board should contain a minimum of 10 feet in water depth under the end of the board. Minimum diving board water depths of 12 feet should exist from six feet back to 20 feet forward of the end of the board—10 to 15 feet between boards, and 12 feet between the board and side of pool.
>
> Special attention should be given to lighting, water temperature, ladders into the pool, acoustical quality and slippery tile on deck areas. Many pools are notoriously deficient in these features. Each of these elements is important for the safety, comfort, and effectiveness of swimming instruction. One hundred foot candlelight is recommended for overhead illumination in an indoor pool. A greater concentration of light is advisable over the end-walls at the shallow and deep ends. Underwater lights add to the appearance of the pool, but are not necessary from a functional perspective. Many pools contain multiple glass side wall panels that reflect on the water surface, and create glare, which can unduly obstruct visual clarity of the swimmer. Glare reflections from the outside should be held to a minimum with an appropriate covering material.
>
> Water temperatures generally range from 78 to 92 degrees, depending upon specific group needs. For example, proficient swimmers prefer cooler temperatures, less than eighty degrees. Handicapped swimmers need water temperatures up to 92 degrees for the development of

relaxation, floating, and modified forms of water propulsion skills. A range of 80–82 degrees is generally acceptable for the safety and comfort of most swimmers. The air temperature should be at least ten degrees above the water temperature to avoid chilling and undue trembling.

Ladders leading into the pool well should be recessed in the side walls. Rungs and grasping handles should not be placed over the side wall into the water since such objects can cause injury to swimmers in outside lanes.

Too often swimming pools, although esthetically constructed, contain hard surfaces of tile, concrete and steel—all of which intensify the echo of sounds. Walls and ceilings should be acoustically treated to allow easy conversation between the instructor and participants. Sound systems simply amplify voices or music, and add to noise pollution when used in untreated acoustical pools.[38]

Checklist for Swimming Pools

The following checklist may be used as a guideline for swimming pools:

General Considerations

- Have cost and time estimates been proposed?
- Is there a clear-cut organizational policy on the purposes and use of the pool?
- Does the design of the pool meet these purposes?
- Does the policy take into consideration any future growth of the organization?
- Has an architect with expertise on swimming pools been consulted on pool design and construction?
- Does the design meet all the standards of the local health authorities?
- Will the pool be limited to employees or is it available for dependents, including small children?
- Will the aquatic fitness instructor be certified in water safety?
- Will the pool be used for competitive events, with seating for spectators?
- Does the policy address the question of use of the pool by local schools and agencies?
- Is there provision for use by the handicapped?

---

38. Personal communication with Doctor John Piscopo. Associate Professor of Physical Education. Department of Physical Therapy and Exercise Science. State University of New York at Buffalo. November, 1987.

Pool Considerations

- Is there adequate overhead clearance and pool depth for diving?
- Is there an effective circulation of water in the pool?
- Is there proper ventilation?
- Is there adequate lighting?
- Is there adequate acoustics?
- Is there proper humidity control?
- Is the deck made of non-slip material?
- Is the bottom of the pool clearly visible at all times?
- Does the pool contain adequate drains?
- Are there daily checks of water temperature, water acidity, chlorine content?
- Is there an office for the instructor with a window overlooking the pool?
- Does the pool office have a telephone in case of emergencies?
- Are there sufficient locker rooms and showers?
- Is there a separate locker room and shower for the instructor?
- Is there provision for lifesaving equipment in case of an accident?
- Have the rules for use of the pool and for diving been prominently displayed?

INDOOR FITNESS EQUIPMENT

Workout or Training Equipment

The following is a list of indoor fitness equipment and purposes for which this equipment may be utilized for fitness programs. Although the list of weight training equipment is ideal and quite extensive, it all could be placed in a room 24 feet × 40 feet.

1. Multi-Purpose Pulley Machine—used for developing the muscles of the legs (by kicking), shoulders, isolated chest and upper arms front and back
2. Mats—used for stretching and calisthenics
3. Treadmill—used for cardiovascular endurance or aerobic conditioning involving the legs. Walking, jogging or running can be performed on this piece of equipment.
4. Bicycle Ergometer—used for cardiovascular endurance or aerobic conditioning

5. Rowing Ergometer—used for cardiovascular endurance or aerobic conditioning

6. Dual Action Bike—used for developing cardiovascular endurance or aerobic conditioning involving the legs and arms

7. Computerized Bicycle—used for developing cardiovascular endurance or aerobic capacity involving the legs

8. Barbells with plates—used for developing muscles of the arms, shoulders, back and legs

9. Dumbbells with rack—used singular or together for developing muscles of the wrists, forearms, upper arms, shoulders, back and, if lying down on a bench, for developing muscles of the chest

10. Inclined Abdominal Board—used for developing muscles of the stomach

11. Thigh and Knee Machine—used for developing the muscles of the upper thighs and knees

12. Leg Curl Machine—used for developing the muscles of the backs of the thighs and sitting muscles

13. Pulley Lat Machine—used for developing muscles of the middle and upper back

14. Combination English Chair and Hyperextension—used for developing muscles of the stomach and lower back

15. Inclined Bench—used with dumbbells for developing muscles of the arms and chest

16. Fly Machine Chair—used for developing isolated muscles of the chest

17. Free Standing Hip Flexor—used for developing muscles of the lower abdomen

18. Weight Training Machine (8 stations)—used for developing muscles of the legs, upper and lower body, abdomen, arms and back

19. Flat Exercise Bench—used with dumbbells for developing muscles of the chest.

Testing Equipment

Some managers, after closely examining the possibilities of having potential participants undergo a physical fitness test and finding there are no outside providers, may then decide to conduct their own testing program. When that is the case, the following equipment is necessary:

- Bench Press—used to measure upper-body strength
- Flexibility Box—used to determine the flexibility of the backs of the thighs
- Leg Press—used to measure lower-body strength
- Skinfold Caliper—used to measure body composition, i.e., lean body weight as compared to fat body weight
- Treadmill—used to evaluate the efficiency of the cardiorespiratory system and to determine exercise prescriptions*
- Vitalograph Spirometer—used to measure vital capacity and forced expiratory volume in one second.

OUTDOOR FACILITIES FOR FITNESS PROGRAMS

Exercise Circuit

When managers begin to investigate the possibility of constructing outdoor fitness facilities for their organizations, what frequently surfaces is an exercise circuit. Other names given to an outdoor fitness facility are exercise trails, fitness trails, or parcourse fitness circuits. An exercise circuit may be purchased from a commercial vendor or it may be constructed locally ("homemade"). These exercise circuits have been designed to improve cardiovascular endurance or aerobic capacity, muscular strength, muscular endurance and flexibility. An exercise circuit may range from one to two miles in length and from four to six feet in width. It contains a series of exercise stations.

"Parcourse" fitness circuits have become popular in recent years, for they combine all the elements for a scientifically designed exercise program. The circuit is composed of eighteen exercise stations and can be used by all levels of exercisers—beginning, intermediate, and advanced. Signs at each station show how to perform each exercise.

Parcourse fitness circuits are unique because at each station there is a "par" system. For example, station number 3 is designated for "toe touches." At the beginner's level, one should attempt to do 5 touches on each side; at the intermediate level, 10 touches to each foot; and at the advanced level, 15 touches to each foot ("par"). In addition to the eighteen exercise stations, there is a jogging path. Some older employees may

---

*Note: A bicycle ergometer may be substituted for the treadmill.

wish to walk through the course and not use the stations, while others may wish to bicycle on the path.[39]

OUTDOOR FITNESS EQUIPMENT

Parcourse Circuit

The exercise stations that comprise a Parcourse fitness circuit are known as outdoor fitness equipment. Each station is designed so as to provide participants with specific types of exercises. The following are the numbers and names of stations included in a typical Parcourse fitness circuit and the purposes:

Number	Name	Purpose
1	Achilles Stretch	— used for developing the muscles of the back of the legs
2	Sit and Reach	— used for stretching the muscles of the back of the thighs and the lower back
3	Touch Toes	— used to warm-up the muscles of the legs and lower back
4	Knee Lift	— used for developing the muscles of the lower abdomen
5	Jumping Jacks	— used predominately for developing the heart muscle but also for muscles of the entire body
6	Log Hop	— used for developing the heart muscle by using the legs
7	Step-Up	— used for developing the heart muscle by using the legs
8	Circle Body	— used for stretching the large body muscles
9	Body Curl	— used for developing the muscles of the lower abdomen
10	Chin-Up	— used for developing the muscles of the upper body, arms and back
11	Hop-Kick	— used for developing the large muscles of the body and also the heart muscle
12	Vault-Bar	— used for developing the muscles of the leg

39. *Portland's Parcourse Fitness Circuit* (Blue Cross/Blue Shield of Maine, Portland, Maine), n.d.

13	Sit-Up	— used for developing the muscles of the upper abdomen
14	Push-Up	— used for developing the muscles of the upper body and chest
15	Bench Leg Raise	— used for developing the muscles of the lower abdomen
16	Hand-Walk	— used for developing the muscles of the upper arms
17	Leg-Stretch	— used for stretching the muscles of the leg
18	Balance-Beam	— used for developing the muscles of the entire body, excluding the heart.

COMMUNITY-BASED FACILITIES

Renting Facilities

When top management makes the decision not to provide on-site facilities for a health and fitness program, an alternative approach that organizations may wish to explore is to rent facilities. However, managers must be prudent in investigating the renting of facilities. Therefore, the following checklist may prove helpful:

Checklist for Renting Facilities

- What is the cost of the facility?
- What is the availability of the facility?
- What is the suitability of the facility in terms of the room(s) and equipment?
- What is the capacity of the facility?
- Is the facility designed for both men and women?
- Is the facility at a convenient location?
- Is there a specific time available for participants or is the facility shared?
- Is the facility available for individual workouts as well as group activities?
- Does the facility have an instructional staff or does the organization renting the facility furnish the staff?

Source: Parcourse Limited, Inc., 444 Clementina Street, San Francisco, CA 94103.

• Does the facility have insurance coverage for injuries or accidents, or does the organization furnish its employees with insurance coverage?

Facilities for Consideration

When managers begin to explore the community-based facilities that may be available, some of the following should be considered:

• Boys and Girls Clubs
• Churches
• Fraternal organizations
• Health Clubs
• High schools, colleges and universities
• Recreational facilities
• YMCA's and YWCA's

Managers should be looking for aerobic exercise rooms, conference or meeting rooms for delivering health education programs, gymnasiums, indoor tracks, men's and women's locker rooms and showers, swimming pools, and weight training rooms.

SUMMARY

Managers need to think in both philosophical and financial terms when organizing facilities and purchasing equipment for a comprehensive health and fitness program. Setting precise standards for facilities and equipment is unrealistic, because organizations vary as to size, number of employees, types of employees, financial resources and newness of health and fitness programs. However, it seemed prudent in this chapter to provide managers with general descriptions of health and fitness facilities and equipment.

For several reasons, on-site facilities are preferred. Therefore, guidelines to assist managers in estimating space requirements are listed. In addition, when organizing facilities and purchasing equipment, managers need to be aware of the many important considerations discussed in this chapter.

Health education facilities are an important part of any health and fitness program. They will vary in sizes and configurations. Health education equipment and their uses are listed.

A discussion of indoor fitness facilities is an integral part of this chapter. Also, some important information on swimming pools is presented.

Indoor fitness equipment is listed as well as its purposes. Types of testing equipment and their purposes are also included.

Outdoor fitness facilities, with a major emphasis on a Parcourse fitness circuit, are discussed, since they are considered beneficial to any health and fitness program.

The chapter is concluded with a discussion of community-based facilities. Although not preferred, they may be an alternative to on-site facilities.

PART IV
LEADING THE HEALTH AND
FITNESS PROGRAM

Chapter VIII

LEADING THE HEALTH
AND FITNESS PROGRAM:
HUMAN RESOURCES

INTRODUCTION

"Leadership," as defined here, is a process of directing staff behavior in order to achieve program goals and objectives. Managers must both assume the leadership role and work closely with the staff if the health and fitness program is to be successful. As pointed out in Chapter II, health and fitness managers are people and service oriented; they work with the staff to form a team to assist participants in realizing their goals and objectives.

It has been said many times that a good manager is a good leader, but a good leader is not necessarily an effective manager. Although health and fitness managers have the right to influence their staff because of the power of the position, they may not opt to exercise this right. The staff may choose to be influenced by other staff members or by varying conditions.[40] For example, a manager of a health and fitness program is responsible for giving directions to a staff; yet, the staff may be influenced by contacts with the in-house physician, the medical consultant, other staff members, or their knowledge of what participants are interested in and actually need.

LEADING THE HEALTH AND FITNESS STAFF

Motivating the Staff for Performance

"Motivating" or leading a staff are terms that are often used synonymously. As a matter of fact, managers may use the same skills and

---

40. Adapted from Silagyi, Jr., *Management*, p. 432.

techniques for either motivating or leading their staffs; for a staff must be motivated in order to achieve the desired goals and objectives.

At this point in the discussion, the following three terms are defined:

- *Motivation* refers to internal psychological conditions identified as inner drives, impulses, or intentions that move a person to behave in a particular manner.
- *Motive* refers to some inner drive, impulse, or intention that moves a person to behave in a certain manner.
- "*Motivating* is a process of moving oneself and others to work toward attainment of individual and organizational objectives."[41]

Ostro provides managers with the following five principles with respect to motivating a staff:

- You must mean what you say and never betray a confidence.
- You must be a staff to lean on.
- You must never compromise the values you are expressing.
- You must never make a promise you cannot keep.
- You must be the kind of person your colleagues . . . would be willing to share a foxhole with.[42]

Although there are several theories on motivation, the one selected for this discussion provides some important information to health and fitness managers. Successful motivation is predicated upon the satisfaction of certain basic needs:

The Basic Needs

Maslow, a well-known psychologist, has developed a theory of motivation that uses a holistic approach which sees all parts or systems of an individual as acting and reacting as one unit. This theory is based on a hierarchy of needs in which an individual progresses from basic needs to self-actualization. The needs at each level must be met (satisfied) before the individual may proceed to the next level.

The Physiological Needs. The physiological needs are those which a person must have to maintain his or her body in such a state as to survive—hunger, thirst and so forth. They are the starting point for

41. Michael H. Meson, Michael Albert and Franklin Khedouri, *Management*, 2nd ed. (New York, NY: Harper and Row, Publishers, 1985), p. 344.

42. Henry Ostro, "How Do You Motivate Your Staff," *Scholastic Coach*, 51:3, 6, October, 1981.

motivation, as they serve as channels for all sorts of other needs as well. If these needs are not met, other (higher) needs may cease to exist. For example, a person who thinks he or she is hungry may really be looking for comfort. A person's outlook for the future will change if one need dominates all others. Moreover, for an extremely dangerous and hungry individual, no other interest exists but food.[43]

The Safety Needs. Once the physiological needs have been met, the safety needs emerge. These include security; stability; dependency; protection; freedom from fear, anxiety, and chaos; need for structure, order, law, limits, strength in the protector and so on. An individual's outlook on life, both current and future, is dependent upon the dominating goal. For example, practically everything looks less important than safety and protection.[44]

The Belongingness and Love Needs. If both the physiological and safety needs have been met, then will follow the need for affection and love and the need to belong. Now the individual will feel keenly the need for friends, a wife or husband and children. He or she strives to attain a place in a group or family and will want more than anything else to have a place in the world, and may even forget he or she once was hungry.

In our society, the lack of fulfillment of these needs is most commonly the cause of maladjustment and pathology. One thing that must be emphasized is that the need for love is not synonymous with sex. Sex is considered a purely physiological need.[45]

The Esteem Needs. All people need a high evaluation of themselves and the respect and esteem of others. They feel the need for both achievement and prestige. A lack of these needs leads to feelings of inferiority and of helplessness, resulting in discouragement and neurotic trends. The most healthy self-esteem derives from *deserved* respect from others, not undeserved adulation.[46]

The Need for Self-Actualization. An artist must paint, a poet must write, a musician must make music. A person must be what he or she must be. The specific need of each person will, of course, vary greatly: ideal mother, great athlete, inventor, for example. These needs

---

43. Abraham H. Maslow, *Motivation and Personality*, 2nd ed. (New York, NY: Harper and Row Publishers, 1970), pp. 35–37.

44. Ibid., p. 39.

45. Ibid., pp. 43–44.

46. Ibid., pp. 45–46.

usually follow prior satisfaction with the physiological, safety, love and esteem needs.[47]

Determining Staff Needs

Individuals who make the decision to become health and fitness professionals and are employed as staff members in an organization have certain needs, the same as any other professionals. Managers should be cognizant of their staff members' needs and assist them in every way possible. Accordingly, the following are central for determining the needs of a health and fitness staff:

Career Goals

Although general goals are discussed in Chapter III, that chapter intentionally omitted career goals. Therefore, career goals are included here because they relate to determining staff needs. Now that the individual is a health and fitness professional, he or she should promptly establish short-term, intermediate, and long-term goals. Career goals should be set in realistic terms, be consistent with the staff member's personal beliefs, self-image, and capabilities and should take into account that person's strengths, weaknesses, experience, interests, values, knowledge of the position, trends in the field of health and fitness, and possible opportunities for professional growth. Two or more staff members can help one another in setting career goals. However, there should be only a few career goals. For example, a health and fitness instructor may strive to become a manager of a comprehensive health and fitness program.

Support

A staff member who is trying to reach his or her career goal(s) needs support from both coworker(s) and the manager. In fact, the manager should encourage support among his or her staff in their attempts at developing their careers. Such support may come by the way of special assignments, temporary changing of positions, in-service training, seminars, conferences and credit courses. Managers need to display an ongoing interest in the work progress of the staff as well as in their future positions within the program and in the profession.

---

47. Ibid., pp. 46–47.

Recognition

Staff members should be recognized for their performance as individuals. The need for recognition is a strong one which should not be overlooked by managers. When possible, it is beneficial to use other people as examples of those who have had successful careers in the field of health and fitness. By so doing, managers help a staff member realize his or her potential. Moreover, the staff member's feelings of self-worth will increase. Recognition, very much a part of all of us, can be used to influence others. It is important that recognition be satisfied in a positive manner so as to prevent problems that can surface when a staff member seeks acknowledgment in negative ways. Recognition is a motivator which managers should use frequently.

Trust and Respect

The need for trust and respect are important to staff members as well as to the manager. Each staff member must live by the principles in which he or she believes in order to gain respect from both participants and coworker(s). Once lost, respect is hard to regain.

If a manager has developed a feeling of trust and respect for the staff, they will open up to him or her. The manager should listen to them intently and with compassion, offering guidance and, if necessary, enlisting help from others.

Direction

Health and fitness staff members need direction; they need to know what managers expect from them. Managers need to get their message across in the right way to their staff. After meeting with their manager, staff members should leave the meeting knowing what part(s) they will play in any plan and what results are expected.

Staff members need to be kept informed of problems, changes, achievements or new policies which will affect them. It is the job of the manager to keep the staff fully informed.

Professional Advancement

The professional advancement of a staff member(s) depends on the growth of the program as well as on the organization's policy on staff development and promotion. As they occur, the manager, through postings, should announce job openings within the staff. Managers should have already prepared a written job description for each position within the program.

After spending much time and effort in developing a good staff, some managers are reluctant to let their staff members move on to bigger and better jobs outside the organization. Therefore, they have a tendency to hoard their good staff members. This action is unprofessional and does not support the career goals of staff members.

Job Satisfaction

"Job satisfaction is the degree to which an individual feels positively or negatively about various aspects of the job, including assigned tasks, the work setting, and relationships with co-workers."[48]

When the job and conditions associated with it meet the expectations of the staff member, satisfaction results. The higher the staff member's satisfaction, the less likely will the staff member be absent or leave the program. Often, a staff member becomes discouraged and frustrated with his or her job and seeks other employment. However, turnover can be lessened if the staff is kept up-to-date on the latest trends in the health and fitness profession. (Also see section, "Developing and Maintaining Satisfaction," further on in this chapter.)

Education and Training

Changes and advances in the health and fitness field make furthering the education and/or training of staff members an absolute necessity. Credit courses at a university or college, in-service training courses, conferences and seminars which focus on a particular relative subject are always welcomed by a staff. Regardless of the type, the program should be made available to the entire staff, not just to specific individuals. These programs can also act as refresher courses to bring staff members up-to-date on new techniques and advances in health and fitness.

Designing Reward Systems

As an introduction to this section, it seems logical to define the term "reward" and the two basic types of rewards. This term has been defined in different ways by several authors in the management field. However,

---

48. John R. Schermerhorn, Jr., *Management For Productivity*, 2nd ed. (New York, NY: John Wiley and Sons, 1986), p. 215.

the definition which follows, selected for this book, seems appropriate: "A reward is anything an individual perceives as valuable."[49]

The two basic types of rewards are known as intrinsic and extrinsic:

> Intrinsic rewards are rewards that are valued in and of themselves. . . . Examples of intrinsic rewards falling into this category are such things as people's feelings of personal competence as a result of performing a job well, feelings of personal accomplishment or achievement associated with attaining a goal or objective, feelings of freedom from direction and personal responsibility arising from being granted autonomy regarding how work activities are to be carried out, and feelings of personal growth and development resulting from success in new and challenging areas of personal endeavor.[50]
>
> Just as intrinsic rewards are internally generated by the person him or herself, extrinsic rewards are externally generated by someone or something else. . . . [51]

Perhaps the best example of an extrinsic reward is money, almost always given to a health and fitness staff as salaries and merit raises. However, in some cases bonuses and profit-sharing plans are also used as extrinsic rewards. Managers should also be cognizant of the fact that extrinsic rewards frequently have a positive impact upon intrinsic motivation.

Reward systems, if they are to be successful, need careful planning and implementation. The manner in which reward systems are designed depends upon the people who make up the staff. Some health and fitness staff members will strive for achievement, while others seek affiliation. Managers will do well to remember that a reward system that works well for one person may not work equally well for another.

Staff members who have a desire for achievement require a reward system which is structured, specific, and performance oriented. Health and fitness personnel work well and are satisfied when rewards are based upon their performance. These persons prefer a monetary-based reward system.

For staff members who seek affiliation, a socially oriented based reward system can suffice. These staffers pursue friendships, status, and close interpersonal relationships with coworkers. They will readily accept any extra assignment socially attractive and satisfying that is given to them

49. Mescon, Albert and Khedouri, *Management*, p. 349.

50. Daniel C. Feldman and Hugh J. Arnold, *Managing Individual and Group Behavior In Organizations* (New York, NY: McGraw-Hill Co., 1983), p. 162.

51. Ibid., p. 163.

by the manager. For the best results, it is recommended that a reward system for health and fitness professionals incorporate both achievement and affiliation. Although some staffers may have a greater need for one or the other, the ideal reward system should include both. The following is a list of guidelines that will make a reward system both attractive to any health and fitness staff and is administratively sound:

- The reward system should be designed to include both achievement (performance) and affiliation (socialization).
- If the reward is given for achievement (performance), the staff member should clearly understand the criteria upon which it is based.
- If the reward is to be an increase in the staff member's salary, the increase must be large enough to satisfy both the staff member's present and future needs; and, of course, that increase must be included in the budget.
- It is important that any monetary reward offered to a staff member(s) be in compliance with the organization's salary policy.
- Whenever an affiliation reward is given to a staff member it should also be acknowledged by both the manager's supervisor and by top management.
- The reward system should be simple and, above all, understandable.
- Managers should design the reward system so as to allow staff members to receive their rewards as soon as possible after having earned them.
- The reward should not be designed so that it is unrealistic. Be certain that once a reward is promised to a staff member, it can be delivered.
- The reward system should be designed so that staff members are required to cooperate with one another.
- The reward system should allow for unavoidable circumstances over which a staff member has no control.
- Above all, one must remember that money may not be considered as great a reward to some as it will be to others. The same is true of affiliation rewards.

Managers need to analyze carefully all the above guidelines prior to designing a reward system. Moreover, changes may be necessary as health and fitness staff members are promoted, leave the program, and/or are added to the staff.

Developing and Maintaining Satisfaction*

Some of the most important attitudes in the work setting are those that relate to one's feelings about the job including the environment surrounding the job—that is job satisfaction. Indeed, job satisfaction has become one of the most common measures of the effectiveness of the organization or a particular program. This is due in part to the fact that high levels of job satisfaction have been related to increased commitment to the organization or program, job involvement, improved physical and mental health, and a heightened quality of work life. Dissatisfaction, on the other hand, is more likely to produce complaints, absence, turnover, and stress with its associated emotional and physical ailments. Job satisfaction is important if for no other reason than most of us devote significantly more of our lives to work than we do to any other activity. One need not be a great humanitarian to accept the argument that this time should be as pleasant as possible.[52]

Concept of Job Satisfaction

While few question the importance of job satisfaction, many confuse it with the term "morale"; indeed, they are often used interchangeably. Job satisfaction refers to the attitudes of a single individual, while morale is used to describe the feelings of a group of employees or a unit.[53]

When one thinks of job satisfaction, it is the job, itself, that immediately comes to mind; that is, the person's feelings, both positive and negative, that flow immediately and directly from doing work—feeling on enjoyment, accomplishment, achievement. In other words, job satisfaction is an internal state, or "intrinsic," or simply feelings the person has about the job as he or she works. There are other components of job satisfaction, as presented in Figure 5, that are "extrinsic" to the job. Stated differently, they comprise the environment surrounding the job such as the behavior of one's boss and coworkers, compensation, working conditions, higher management, and organizational policy. Unlike intrinsic job satisfaction (e.g., the feeling that I succeed on this task), extrinsic satisfaction arises from the actions of others. It was my boss who unfairly criticized my work, for example, or he/she gave me a pay raise, or it is the support and friendship expressed by my coworkers. All are sources

---

*This section was written by Doctor Charles Greene, Professor of Management, School of Business, Economics and Management, University of Southern Maine, Portland, Maine.

52. Charles N. Greene, Everett E. Adam, Jr., and Ronald J. Ebert, *Management* (Englewood Cliffs, NJ: Prentice-Hall, 1985), pp. 115–116.

53. David J. Cherrington, *Organizational Behavior* (Boston, MA: Allyn and Bacon, 1989), p. 306.

Figure 5

The Job and the Environment Surrounding the Job

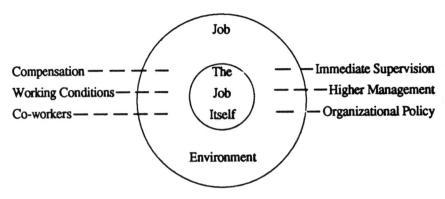

of satisfaction, but they arise from others and not from the individual, him- or herself.

Developing Satisfaction

Clearly, satisfaction starts with the job. Work, itself, must at least meet some minimal standards of employee interest and feelings of being worthwhile. However, beyond this point, the individual must feel adequately satisfied with the extrinsic components, the conditions surrounding the job, before much more can be done to enhance satisfaction with the job. For example, consider the following illustrations:

• **Compensation.** Pay levels must be sufficient and equitable; that is, pay should reflect market values and be equivalent to comparable jobs both within the organization and at similar organizations in the community.

• **Conditions of Work.** While individuals vary in terms of what they consider desirable working conditions, the most obvious action here is the removal of the most severe problems or barriers to a pleasant work environment (e.g., three staff people crowded into a small office).

• **Coworkers.** Perhaps the most common problem involving coworkers are status and/or reward systems that encourage competition where cooperation is needed. Such individual incentives need to be reduced and group incentives that recognize interdependence among group members developed.

• **Immediate Supervision.** The boss's behavior toward a subordinate clearly has significant bearing on the subordinate's satisfaction. Among those traits that are valued most are honesty, fairness, and relevant expertise.

• **Higher Management and Organizational Policy.** Both of these conditions of the job environment unfortunately are seen by employees as sources of dissatisfaction—e.g., insensitive and the "there's no damn reason for doing it but policy requires it" or obsolete policies. An administrator along with peers can often overcome or alleviate policy problems and appropriately shield subordinates from an insensitive management.

Once major sources of dissatisfaction have been removed from the job environment (or, stated differently, the employee is at least relatively satisfied with the extrinsic components), then much more can be done to enhance satisfaction with the job. Two of the most important actions an administrator can take involve work, itself, and delegation. The former concerns assignment of tasks or modification of existing tasks that the employee particularly values or that are more consistent with employee interests. The latter involves ideally delegating an entire block of work, a major assignment, for which the employee assumes total or primary accountability and which he or she can "work through" from its inception to successful completion. Although they are beyond the scope of this book, another set of actions that can be taken require redesign of the employee's job. For example, "increasing the variety of tasks for which the employee is responsible, establishing feedback mechanisms that place quality control under the employee's own control, and combining tasks so that the employee is no longer responsible for a single, usually boring task, but rather several related tasks that comprise a whole job.[54] Not all employees will respond favorably to such job efforts, however. Some may not desire the bigger job that inevitably evolves.

In-Service Training

Webster's New World Dictionary defines the word "in-service" as "designating or of training, as in special courses, workshops, etc., given to employees in connection with their work to help them develop skills,

---

54. For further discussion of job redesign programs, the reader should note J.R. Hackman, G. Oldham, and K. Purdy, "A New Strategy for Job Enrichment," *California Management Review,* 17, Summer, 1975, pp. 55–71. Additional information is provided in varying detail in most college level management and organizational behavior texts.

etc."[55] In-service training is usually given at the site of the health and fitness program. In-service training programs are offered separately to health educators and fitness personnel. They are different from academic learning because the training is more flexible and individualized. Programs such as these focus on applied knowledge and are aimed at the two specific positions within the program.

Managers of health and fitness programs have an obligation to provide in-service training because it is an investment in the future. Such training may be led by the manager, if he or she has the expertise, or by a facilitator from the outside. Often, the training methods utilized are specially designed to keep the staff's interest at a high level. Before implementing an in-service program, the manager should clearly define goals and objectives so that the expected outcome is understood by all staff personnel. All in-service training should contain two kinds of objectives: learning and behavioral. Learning objectives are defined as those that the staff should know upon completion of the program, whereas behavioral objectives are stated as how well staffers will perform at the end of an in-service program. The following suggested principles for designing in-service programs may prove helpful:

- Evaluate the background and experience of the staff and provide for their input into what may be needed.
- Define the goals and objectives of the program.
- Design the program to meet the goals and objectives, including cost and time away from the job.
- Conduct the program.
- Write an evaluation of the program's strength and weaknesses and recommendations for changes, if any.[56]

According to Famularo, the person conducting the in-service training program may use any one or a combination of the following methods:

- Lectures—Frequently used as a training method because it can bring a staff up to a satisfactory level of knowledge, skills and techniques. Lectures may include a variety of educational media and materials such as slides, slide tapes, films, transparencies and videocassettes.

---

55. David B. Guralnik, Editor in Chief, *Webster's New World Dictionary*, Second College Edition (New York, N.Y., Prentice-Hall Press, 1986), p. 728.

56. Personal communications with Doctor John Bay, former Dean, School of Business, Economics and Management, University of Southern Maine, Portland, Maine, January, 1989.

- Discussion Groups—Dividing the staff into health educators and fitness personnel, staff members may learn by hearing from other members regarding what they have found helpful in their day-to-day experiences. In some cases, discussion groups may be as effective as the lecture method.
- Role Playing—May be utilized for the actual playing out of roles between a staff member and a participant. Staff members develop their own dialogue spontaneously as they go along and call for a staff member to participate actively. If the situation is taped and played back to the staff, they may review and critique the performance. This setting allows the staff member to view how his or her behavior may affect the participant.
- Games—The use of games as a method for in-service training has merit. Games can be utilized to give a staff member the feeling of being in control. Through the use of games, staffers can be taught the importance of cooperation. Games may also be used as a motivator.
- Behavior Modeling—This method of in-service training is perhaps best suited for fitness professionals. The staff member learns by having the skill demonstrated. He or she in turn practices what has been observed. To be effective, the skill is rehearsed, feedback given, and then transferred to actual practice on the job.
- Cases—A case study is another method that may be used for in-service training. Case studies are written descriptions of hypothetical or actual situations that exist in a health and fitness program. When this method is utilized, it can help staff members sharpen their analytical skills, exchange ideas, and develop principles and concepts which can be applied to the position.[57]

From the above information, managers should have some idea of ways of providing an in-service training program to health and fitness professionals. Regardless of education and experience, through in-service training all staff personnel can gain a valuable body of knowledge that focuses directly on their positions. Again, it's the manager who should plan and organize this program.

Career Stages, Development and Planning

Health and fitness professionals who possess a post-secondary education are seeking meaningful jobs, increased personal freedom, and better opportunities, in addition to demanding input in matters that affect them. They are deeply concerned about their careers, as a satisfying

---

57. Adapted from Joseph J. Famularo, Editor, *Handbook of Human Resources Administration*, 2nd ed. (New York, NY: McGraw-Hill Book Co., 1986), pp. 29–30.

career is an important part of a person's working life. Once on a job, staff member(s) should develop a basic understanding of careers. This kind of information may also help managers. But before continuing with this discussion, the topics "career stages," "career development," and "career planning" are explained.

Individuals go through distinct but interrelated stages in their careers. The simplest version would include four stages:

1. Prework stage: attending school
2. Initial work stage: moving from job to job
3. Stable work stage: maintaining one job
4. Retirement stage: leaving active employment.[58]

These four stages are briefly explained below:

> Stage I: Young professionals enter an organization with technical knowledge, but not with understanding of the organization's demand and expectations. . . .
>
> Stage II: Once through the dependency of Stage I, the professional employee moves into a stage which calls for working independently. Passage of this stage depends upon proven competence in some specific technical area. . . .
>
> Stage III: Professionals in Stage III are expected to become the mentors of those in Stage I. They also tend to broaden their interests and deal more and more with people outside the organization. . . .
>
> Stage IV: Some professional employees remain in Stage III, while others progress to yet another stage which involves shaping the direction of the organization itself. . . . [59]

The above four career stages are most fitting for professionals who are employed in a health and fitness program; only the term "organization" needs to be replaced by the term "program."

"Career development" is the planning of an individual's career that includes education, training, quest for positions and procurement, and work experiences. From the perspective of a health and fitness program, it is a process of guiding the placement, movement, and growth of a staff member through performance evaluation, planned activities, and planned position steps within a health and fitness program.

"Career planning" involves matching an individual's career aspirations with the opportunities available in an organization.[60] This includes evaluating one's strengths and weakness, setting career goals, investi-

---

58. Donnelly, Gibson and Ivancevich, *Fundamentals*, p. 703.

59. Ibid., pp. 704–706.

60. Ibid., p. 770.

gating career opportunities, and developing a career path within the program and in other such programs.

Health and fitness managers play the role of counselors in career planning because in most cases staffers need help and advice when planning their careers. The counseling is usually part of the individual's performance evaluation. The fact remains, however, that the ultimate responsibility for career planning rests with each staff member, not with the manager.

MANAGEMENT OF THE HEALTH AND FITNESS OFFICE

Importance Of Office Management

It seems fair to say that management of the health and fitness office has received relatively little attention by managers. This lack of attention on the part of managers can be attributed to several reasons: lack of understanding as to how the office should function, lack of office management education training, lack of time available for supervising the office and its personnel. Yet, potential participants who wish to register for any of the health and/or fitness programs make their initial contacts through the office. If their first impression of the office is that it is well-run and efficiently managed, so too will they consider the program(s). On the other hand, if they perceive that the office is poorly run and disorganized, they will think the same about the program(s).

Every health and fitness manager needs to know, and understand, the essentials of office management. Whether a large comprehensive program, one or two health programs, or one or two fitness programs are offered, the need for effective office management is very important. Furthermore, regardless of whether there is no secretary or office equipment available, the same functions must be performed. Moreover, the size of the program does not change the internal requirements of the office, only the work volume. Typing, filing, maintaining records, duplicating, placing phone calls, answering the phone, and so forth are all an integral part of a successful program. In a small health and fitness program, the manager must perform many of the office functions; whereas in a large comprehensive program, these functions are performed by trained office personnel.

The work of the manager and the staff is greatly assisted by the secretary, since staff members are relieved of a variety of responsibilities that can be much better performed by trained office personnel. Obviously, health and fitness professionals are not trained to do office work. When a trained secretary is employed, communications to participants and others in the organization are significantly enhanced.

In a health and fitness office, there are correct and incorrect ways of performing all of the office functions. Of course, performing them correctly saves time and money. The health and fitness office must function smoothly, efficiently, and effectively if the program(s) is to be popular and, therefore, successful. Consequently, all office procedures must have been tested and proven before they are implemented. A good way to gather tested and proven health and fitness office procedures is to request them from several other small or large program offices. Managers must not forget that the health and fitness office and its personnel need to be considered an extremely important part of the program(s).

Functions of the Office

Like any other type of office, a health and fitness office is set up to carry out specific functions; therefore, the size of the office will vary according to the extensiveness of the program(s). In many small organizations, the manager is fortunate to have his or her own office; often, he or she has to share an office with another manager. On the other hand, some large organizations that have many participants in various programs require a large health and fitness office. In these situations, a large office is absolutely necessary to accommodate the office personnel and all the latest types of equipment. For example, an office such as this may include (in addition to general office equipment, such as a telephone, a typewriter, a desk, a chair, and a file cabinet) a copying machine, a portable dictating machine, and a computer.

Following is a list of functions performed in a health and fitness office. These functions, common to any size office, will be briefly discussed below.

• Placing Calls and Answering the Telephone

If the health and fitness program is large enough, a secretary is employed, full-time, for the office. This person places calls and answers the telephone. Of course, if a full-time secretary is not employed because of the number of programs being offered, these functions may be performed by a part-time secretary or by the manager, if the secretary is absent. Regardless of the situation, the telephone should be answered promptly, professionally, courteously, and in a friendly and helpful manner. When answering the phone, the individual should identify the program and give his or her name. For example, "Health and Fitness Program. Vicki (or Bill) speaking. May I help you?" It is important that a pen and message pad be available at all times and that a procedure be developed for promptly transmitting the message to the appropriate person.

When telephone calls are for the manager and he or she is not available, there need to be some guidelines for the secretary to follow as to the desired information that should be given out. If the manager is meeting in his or her office, there needs to be an understanding with the secretary regarding being interrupted. Furthermore, the secretary should know where the manager is at all times during working hours; that is, at meetings, appointments, lunch, is ill, on vacation and so forth. When calls are made and staff members are not available, the secretary should always ask to take a message. If the caller doesn't wish to leave a message, request that he or she give his or her name and ask this question, "May I have Mrs. Ross or Mr. Langford return your call?" The telephone is an important instrument for communication and should be used in a professional manner at all times.

- **Filing**

A health and fitness office, like any other professional office, cannot function unless it contains one or more metal filing cabinets that are used solely for vertical filing. Furthermore, the files need to be placed so that they are easily accessible for quick reference so as to avoid delays and save time. Filing systems will vary according to the nature of the office; however, for a health and fitness office, the files should contain materials such as survey results, participants' records, reports, staff resumes, job descriptions, correspondence, financial records, purchase order requisitions, copies of rules, procedures and policies, invoices, budgets, charts, minutes of staff meetings, and content of programs.

A filing system for a health and fitness office may be organized in several different ways. The most common and frequently used is alphabetical filing. When utilizing alphabetical filing, no cross-index or list of files is necessary. However, filing by either name, category or program, in addition to alphabetical billing, has proven successful in many health and fitness offices.

Filing by color code has also been used in some health and fitness offices as a quick reference to programs. Each program offered is given a different-colored stripe which is already on the top of the self-sticking label. The last name, then first name, of a participant who is in a particular program is typed under the colored stripe and filed alphabetically. Each participant's folder should contain his or her complete records. Obviously, folders of employees who are in fitness programs contain more materials than those who are in health education programs because of the various forms and records necessary.

Regardless of what filing system is utilized, the system selected must be effective. Furthermore, secretaries must keep their filing up-to-date. Sometimes when secretaries are busy, they have a tendency to leave a considerable amount of material unfiled. This is a poor practice. Managers should remind the secretary that filing needs to be done on a daily basis, if possible.

• Receiving Prospective Participants

Usually the first person a prospective participant comes into contact with is the secretary. It is a good practice for this person to remember employees, keep track of their files, and check with them after they have registered. Furthermore, the secretary should be caring and cheerful. It is important that office personnel are courteous and helpful in answering questions regarding the program(s) that are currently being offered or planned for the near future. The first impression prospective participants get from a visit to a health and fitness office is one that is lasting. It is absolutely necessary then that a health and fitness office have a pleasant atmosphere and demonstrate a sense of people working together and enjoying the work. All prospective participants should be greeted cordially. If they have an appointment to see the manager or a staff person, they should be given a comfortable seat and provided with health and fitness reading materials.

• Corresponding

All health and fitness managers should establish the policy that all correspondence, whether memoranda within the organization or letters going outside, should be answered the same day they are received. Of course, this may not always be possible; but it is a sound practice to attempt to answer correspondence expeditiously. All correspondence should be prepared carefully, using proper grammar, and in a neat manner to meet the highest standards of the secretarial profession. If the manager has to do his or her own correspondence, these same standards apply.

All correspondence should be proofread in order to detect any mistakes. For letters going outside the organization, the address as well as the zip code should be checked for accuracy. Carbon copies should be made for all correspondence and filed under the headings "correspondence inside" or "correspondence outside" for future reference.

At least one full-time secretary for most health and fitness offices may suffice; however, if a full-time secretary is not possible, perhaps a part-time secretary can be employed. If neither a full-time nor part-time secretary is financially possible, perhaps a secretary in some other department can handle the manager's correspondence.

The use of dictaphones can save the health and fitness manager much valuable time. Memoranda and letters may be dictated at any time during the day, night, or over weekends. Thus, the dictated materials will be ready for the secretary to type. Some managers prefer the first draft to be a rough copy, which will be corrected; others prefer that they be only one final copy. When the manager is using the dictaphone, he or she should not be interrupted; it is difficult to compose various correspondences when interruptions occur.

- **Copying Materials**

Making copies of some of the materials that are produced in a health and fitness office is an absolute necessity. In contemporary times there are many kinds of copiers. The manager and secretary should select one that best suits the needs of the office. While some managers believe it is necessary to make duplicate copies of all materials, others feel that only selected materials need to be duplicated. If all office materials are not copied, the question arises as to which of the materials should be copied. Definitely, all memoranda going inside the organization and all letters going outside the organization must have copies. In addition, it is believed that copies should be made of survey results, rules, procedures and policies, financial records, job descriptions, reports, staff resumes, various charts, content of programs, purchase order requisition invoices, and budgets. Making copies of the participants' records seems to be a waste of time and paper. However, because they are almost impossible to replace, it is extremely important that these records never get misplaced or lost.

- **Making Appointments**

The scheduling of a meeting or an engagement is called an appointment. Making and keeping appointments is another function of a health and fitness office. All managers and staff members must make appointments; therefore, it is necessary that a system be developed to remind them of these engagements. The reminder should become a daily routine and will prove helpful, in that no appointments are overlooked or forgotten. Managers will need to meet with other department heads, their supervisors, and groups of potential participants, while staff members will need to make appointments to talk with participants. Furthermore, there will be times when staff members will need to make appointments to talk to the manager. Whatever system is adopted, the secretary must be involved. It is this person's responsibility to see that the manager and the staff members meet their obligations. Moreover, they should not be late or miss an appointment or forget the purpose of the meeting. Secretaries should keep an appointment book on their desks, while managers and staff members need to keep pocket appointment books. To assure accuracy, both of these appointment books must contain identical information. Of course, if no secretary is available, the manager and the staff members must keep their own schedule for appointments. It is a serious mistake for them to rely on their memories.

• Providing Services to Staff

If there are one or more full-time or part-time staff members employed in the health and fitness program, these person(s) can be provided with various services as a function of the office. These services may include typing letters, programs, updates, records, reports, speeches, and participants' records. In addition, the office person may schedule appointments for staff members. When the office does not have a secretary, staffers may, as a last resort, seek assistance in some other office within the organization. This practice is not recommended. A health and fitness program requires a special type of secretary, and typing is not included in a staff member's job description. Furthermore, if a staff member does his or her own typing, time from actual instruction will be taken. Without a full-time or part-time secretary, a health and fitness office cannot function effectively.

The Health and Fitness Secretary

As stated previously, organizations that have health and fitness programs usually employ either a full-time or a part-time secretary, depending on the size of the program. This person is critical to the program.

Although there are promotional steps associated with the secretarial profession, the discussion that follows will focus only on the position of secretary. It would be preferable that these persons have some knowledge of health and fitness. If not, they should acquire, at an early date, an interest in the field and keep themselves reasonably well informed about it.

There are various desirable qualities to look for when hiring secretaries: They should have a well-groomed appearance, a pleasant voice and manner, and a positive and helpful attitude. They should also be courteous, tactful, and reliable. In addition to good basic writing and verbal skills, it would be helpful for the health and fitness secretary to be competent in the use of a portable dictating machine and a word processor.

A study of secretarial competencies, conducted at the University of Southern Maine, revealed that there are "competencies" which effective secretaries should possess. These competencies are divided into four major areas and are most appropriate for health and fitness secretaries. The major areas and their respective competencies are listed here:

Competencies

INTELLECTUAL
- Diagnostic Skill*
- Divergent Thinking*

ENTREPRENEURIAL
- Values Quality and Efficiency*
- Initiative*
- Thinking Ahead and Optimizing

INTERPERSONAL
- Use of Multiple Influence Strategies*
- Interpersonal Sensitivity*
- Helping Orientation

MATURATIONAL
- Job Commitment*
- Sense of Responsibility
- Concern for Image
- Strong Self-Concept
- Assertiveness*
- Grace Under Pressure

The results of the study indicated eight optimal competencies which distinguished the outstanding secretaries. The six remaining required competencies appeared with approximately equal frequency. These required competencies are considered as minimal for effective secretarial work.[61]

Such a secretary is not produced overnight but is the product of years of experience and on-the-job learning. As for education:

---

*Optimal competencies.

61. Freda Bernotavicz and Miriam Clasby, *Competency Across the Campus: The University Secretary* (Portland: Division of Employee Relations, University of Southern Maine, 1984), pp. 2–3.

Secretarial training ranges from high school vocational education programs that teach office practices, shorthand, and typing to 1- to 2-year programs in secretarial science offered by business schools, vocational-technical institutes, and community colleges.[62]

Health and fitness secretaries are more than persons responsible for answering the phone, typing, and filing records. Because of the nature of health and fitness programs, these secretaries need to possess an array of competencies and skills in order to be effective.

Financial Records of Programs

Efficient management of a health and fitness program will necessitate the keeping of financial records for each program that is being offered. This record includes information regarding the income, if any, and the expenditures which are necessary to determine the net cost of each program being conducted. Whether or not a charge is made to employees, the cost must be measured in terms of meeting the health and fitness goals and objectives of the program.

Records make checking the financial status of each program on a quarterly, semiannual, and annual basis possible. Moreover, comparisons can be made with similar health and fitness programs offered by other organizations. Financial records are extremely important for developing a budget. Such records will provide the manager, as well as his or her supervisors, with pertinent information as to the financial status of each program and whether or not the program should continue. Very few, if any, organizations will allow a health and fitness program to continue for any length of time if it runs into a deficit. Health and fitness programs are initiated if there is a need, if they are financially feasible, and if a sufficient number of employees become participants. Financial records then become essential because the manager needs to know the cost of each program that is offered, where the money comes from, and whether the program pays for itself, makes a profit, or goes into deficit.

Establishing a system for maintaining the financial records of health and fitness programs is one responsibility that a manager cannot afford to overlook. If the health and fitness office has a computer, these financial records are maintained there for up to two years and then put into the archives with the supporting documents. If, on the other hand, a computer is not available, financial records must be kept in a suitable file cabinet.

---

62. *Occupational Outlook Handbook,* 1986–87 ed., Bulletin 2250 (Washington, DC: U.S. Dept. of Labor, Bureau of Labor Statistics, April, 1986), p. 282.

Participants' Records

Managers with vision foresee the wisdom of maintaining participants' records, for these records are valuable to both the participant and the manager. If the organization has a medical department, health records are maintained in that office or in the nurse's office. If the organization has neither a medical office nor a nurse's office and is offering health programs, fitness programs, or both, then obviously health records are kept in the manager's office.

Most organizations require their employees to have a pre-employment medical examination. These records are strictly confidential, since they contain personal and family health histories which reveal pre-existing conditions which may or may not affect the work of an employee. Also, if the employee has been injured on the job, the injury should be noted on his or her health record.

If the employee registers in either a health or a fitness program or both, the manager should get permission to review his or her pre-employment medical examination record. It is critical that managers know the health and medical backgrounds of their program participants so that they may better understand the present health status of each participant.

Managers should be mindful that keeping accurate records can be beneficial to both the participants and themselves. For the participants, these records will indicate what health programs they have taken and the duration, month, and year. From a manager's perspective, health records will show names of participants, the programs they have registered for and the dates, the length of time they stayed in the programs, and whether or not they have repeated a program.

Because of confidentiality, pre-employment medical examination records cannot be duplicated. Therefore, managers, with assistance from full-time or part-time health instructors or resource personnel, should keep accurate health records of each participant. Of course, these records are kept in the secretary's office, if available, or in the manager's office. These kinds of records are quite simple and include the participant's name, age, sex, the name of the program, program location, date enrolled, duration, and instructor.

Fitness records are similar to, but differ from, health records, in that they show progress, which can be used for motivation. If the participant has a problem, a record may be helpful in tracking and compiling data.

Participants in fitness programs usually maintain their own records and should keep them up-to-date.

Follow-Up Procedures

No health and fitness program can be called successful unless it has clear-cut follow-up procedures. Actually, there are three follow-up procedures that have proven successful over the years: The first procedure is sending a questionnaire to all participants immediately after the completion of the program. The second procedure is telephoning each participant asking him or her specific pertinent questions. The third procedure is retesting participants who are currently enrolled in fitness programs in order to determine whether or not they have made any progress regarding their physical fitness level.

SUMMARY

The obvious fact is that managers can motivate or lead their staff in such a way that staffers may achieve their goals and objectives. Maslow, a well-known psychologist, developed a theory of motivation using a holistic approach to cause the individual to act and react as one unit. His theory of motivation is one that health and fitness managers should familiarize themselves with.

Because health and fitness professionals have specific needs, managers should assist them in any way possible to meet these needs. Staff needs are discussed in this chapter, all of significant importance.

Regardless of where and what people do for work, they appreciate being rewarded. Intrinsic and extrinsic rewards are defined and examples of each given.

Developing and maintaining job satisfaction among a health and fitness staff is vital if the program is to be successful. Many confuse job satisfaction with "morale" and they are often used interchangeably. But job satisfaction refers to the attitudes of a single individual, while morale is used to describe the feelings of a group of employees of a unit.

Managers have an obligation to provide in-service training and should view such training as an investment in the future. All in-service training contains two kinds of objectives: learning and behavioral.

Health and fitness professionals are no different from other professionals in their concern with their careers. Four career stages are briefly explained as well as career development and career planning.

The importance of office management cannot be taken lightly. Managers need to know and understand the essentials of office management, regardless of whether the health and fitness program is large or small. A health and fitness office is set up to carry out specific functions. These office functions are identified and discussed.

The section on the health and fitness secretary is one that contains some pertinent information. Without this person, the program will be in trouble. Discussed are the secretarial competencies that all effective secretaries should possess.

Keeping financial records of a health and fitness program is a major responsibility. These records make checking on the financial status of each program possible. Therefore, it is the manager's responsibility to set up a system for maintaining financial records, as top management will want to keep track of the fiscal status of the program.

The chapter concludes with a discussion of participant records and follow-up procedures. Both health and fitness participant records are absolutely necessary when these types of programs are being offered. Furthermore, these records must be kept accurately by the secretary (if available), the manager, and the participant.

Chapter IX

LEADING THE HEALTH
AND FITNESS PROGRAM:
FINANCIAL CONSIDERATIONS AND MARKETING

INTRODUCTION

Regardless of the size and type of an organization, managers of health and fitness programs need to spend a fair amount of time on financial considerations and on marketing. Stress on both these areas is essential if the program is to be successful. Consequently, financial considerations and marketing will be discussed in this chapter and will, hopefully, provide some helpful information.

The fiscal responsibility for health and fitness programs rests solely with managers, who are accountable to their immediate supervisors. Managers must establish procedures of financial accountability which conform to the organization's financial policy. Regardless of the program's funding, keeping track of all expenditures and, if appropriate, any revenues associated with the program is of vital importance. Of course, an available secretary can be of tremendous help to the manager. It should be noted that the manner in which health and fitness programs are financed is a strong factor in determining the success of such programs.

CONSIDERING FEES FOR A HEALTH AND FITNESS PROGRAM

How are Fees Determined?

The process involved in determining fees for a health and fitness program may be time consuming. Regardless of whether or not the program is comprehensive in scope, if the organization has such a policy, each health component and/or each fitness component can be given a fee. When managers gather the responses to the questions below, they should have a good grasp as to determining fees.

159

- Is the organization profit or not-for-profit?
- Have the direct and indirect expenses been calculated?
- Have other similar organizations with similar programs been contacted in an effort to compare fees?
- Are the programs fully subsidized by the organization or are the programs offered on a cost-share basis?
- If the programs are on a cost-share basis, will the employee have to pay the full amount for a program if it is not completed?
- Is the fee structure the same for health programs as it is for fitness programs?
- What is the margin of profit if on a profit basis?
- If fees are assessed, are they paid prior to entrance into a program(s) or at any time throughout the duration of a program(s)?
- What is the present and anticipated future financial status of the organization, region, state, and country?
- How often is the fee structure reviewed and evaluated?

When managers analyze the responses to the above questions, they will undoubtedly conclude that the answers will not only vary but also, in some cases, vary substantially. Organizations that have a health and fitness program will have to determine their own fee structure, as there are no set standards for determining fees of health or fitness programs.

Who Determines the Fee Structure?

There seems to be a misconception as to who determines the fees for health programs and/or fitness programs in organizations that have a fee structure. Some people believe that setting up a fee structure is the sole responsibility of the managers. In some cases this may be true. But whenever possible, managers should not act alone in setting fees. A committee composed of the health and fitness staff and, in some cases, the secretary should establish the proposed fee structure. Of course, the manager will have the final say, as they have fiscal responsibility for program(s). Also, it should be said that fees for health programs and/or fitness programs should be reviewed at least annually.

Once the committee is established, there should be frequent meetings held to discuss every financial expenditure associated with a particular program and all revenue, if appropriate. Once this committee has reached a decision regarding fees for programs, the final step is for managers to take the proposed fee structure to their immediate supervisors for approval.

If approved, the fees are now ready to be implemented; if not approved, the fee structure committee must meet again to review the supervisor's recommendations and revise the fee structure accordingly.

FINDING OTHER FINANCIAL RESOURCES

Sooner or later managers of health and fitness programs conducted in various types of organizations will be seeking additional funding. Regardless of the manner in which the program is presently funded, additional funding is always welcome and can be utilized in a variety of ways; namely, for new programs, additional staff, supplies, equipment, facilities and/or rental fees, if appropriate.

Total funding for any health and fitness program may come from organizations (either fully, subsidized or cost-shared), participants (either fully, subsidized or cost-shared), and outside sources or any combination of the above three.

With reference to programs conducted in work places, O'Donnell and Ainsworth state:

> Most funds come directly or indirectly from the employer or employees, but there is some hope that insurance companies, government, and foundations may at least provide short-term financing for such programs. Outside sources of funding will arise as the concept of health promotion in the work place becomes better established.[63]

Managers may also raise additional financial resources by sponsoring special events such as health fairs, nutrition days, walk-a-thons, swim-a-thons, bike-a-thons, aerob-a-thons, danca-thons, employee fitness days, and road races. Naturally, sponsoring special events takes time and effort, but this can be a unique learning experience for novice managers. In the long run, sponsoring special events can not only bring in additional funds but also give more visibility to a health and fitness program.

---

63. Michael P. O'Donnell and Thomas H. Ainsworth, *Health Promotion in the Workplace* (New York, NY: John Wiley and Sons, 1984), p. 534.

MARKETING THE HEALTH AND FITNESS PROGRAM

What is Marketing?

Marketing is a term that has been evolving over the years and that is being extensively used in the business world. Marketing has been called a science and an art. Within recent years, it is being used in the health and fitness field. Health and fitness programs, regardless of what organizations are delivering them and who the participants are, is in actuality a business, whether for-profit or not-for-profit. Managers would be well advised, therefore, to learn as much as possible about marketing and the effect it can have on a health and fitness program.

Two definitions of marketing are mentioned, the first with a total focus on business. The American Marketing Association, representing marketing professionals in the United States and Canada, puts forth the following definition: "Marketing is the process of planning and executing the conception, pricing, promotion, and distribution of ideas, goods, and services to create exchanges that satisfy individual and organizational objectives."[64] The second definition of marketing has been modified so that it applies more closely to health and fitness programs: Marketing is a combination of activities required to direct the flow of programs and services from an organization to the participant in a form, place, time, and at a price that is best able to satisfy participants' needs.

In our contemporary society, marketing a health and fitness program is a must regardless of its delivery base. Moreover, without marketing even an excellent program may have to be compromised.

Understanding the Marketing Process

Very few, if any, organizations that offer health and fitness programs have a marketing manager, although marketing experts have been used as consultants. Regardless of the situation or the size of the program, health and fitness managers should have a basic understanding of the marketing process. Below, five major elements that comprise the marketing process are discussed with responses to five key questions that are related to the major elements of marketing:

---

64. "A.M.A. Board Approves New Marketing Definition," *Marketing News,* 19:1, March, 1985.

Target Audience

The first question is, Who gets the health and/or fitness program? It is important to distinguish between the various ages and the health and/or fitness status of potential participants and to determine what type of program they are interested in pursuing. If potential participants have health problems, are they mild, moderate or severe? Are they remediable? Do they require rehabilitation exercise programs or just regular fitness programs? Another point to keep in mind is that if the target audience is relatively small, the cost of offering the program is prohibitive.

Depending upon the type of organization, target audiences will, of course, vary. If the organization is a work place—business, industry, college, university, hospital, or government agency—it is obvious that all employees, including top, middle and lower management personnel, comprise the target audience. YMCA's, YWCA's, health clubs, and fitness clubs may have as their target audience one or any combination of the following categories: youth, adults, older adults and families. It is important that managers first determine who the target audience is that they wish to reach, then focus upon that particular group(s).

Price

The second question is, How much do the participants have to pay for a health and/or fitness program? As mentioned previously, both direct and indirect costs of each health and fitness program must be calculated before the final price can be determined. The issue of whether the organization is for-profit or not-for-profit is major in determining the price. Another factor to consider is the economics and local conditions at the time the price is being determined.

The optimal price that participants should pay for each health and/or fitness program is a complex issue and one that has no immediate resolution. However, committees and managers should take into account the following when setting participant prices for health and/or fitness programs:

- Identification of all costs, not just cash costs to participants
- Impact of price on motivation level of participants
- Impact of price on desire to enroll

- Impact of price on the composition of the group (such as income level or position in the organizational hierarchy)
- Minimal total revenue required from participants to support the program[65]

Product

The third question is, What does the "product" look like? For the purpose of this book, the product is a comprehensive health and fitness program which should improve the overall health of participants because of its holistic approach. Perhaps the best answer to the above question is to name all the components of the program. It seems logical to divide the components into health and fitness, although they are closely interrelated. A brief description of all the components, environmental management, nutrition and weight management, smoking cessation, stress management, and substance abuse: alcohol and drugs, may be found in Chapter IV. The names of eight fitness components are briefly described under their appropriate categories:

Cardiovascular Endurance

Aerobic dance, aerobic exercise, aquatic fitness and walk/jog.

Muscular Strength and Muscular Endurance

Weight training and timed calisthenics.

Flexibility

Static stretching.

Rehabilitation

Cardiac, pulmonary, low back.

Managers would be well-advised to know and completely understand their product. It is they who have the responsibility of "selling" the program to top management (where appropriate) and to potential participants.

Place

The fourth question is, How does the program get to the participants? The location of health and/or fitness programs will vary according to the organization. The ideal situation is the organization's own facilities used

---

65. O'Donnell and Ainsworth, *Health Promotion*, p. 562.

to accommodate both health education and fitness programs; moreover, health education facilities are usually available in most organizations. Once health and fitness programs have been developed and are ready to be implemented, how these get to the participants becomes a simple matter. If organizations have on-site facilities, programs can be delivered easily and conveniently. But, on the other hand, if organizations do not have their own facilities, managers are forced to look elsewhere. The problem of not having facilities is that many work place organizations at the present time have not made a financial commitment. When organizations do not have the necessary facilities but do have a health and fitness program, they must look for a facility for potential participants. Some of the options open to these organizations are to have a facility built, or, if not feasible, to borrow, rent, or share an existing facility within the community.

Promotion

The fifth and last question is, How is the health and fitness program "sold" to top-level management and to the current and potential participants? The answer is to "sell" the program to top-level management in organizations in terms of benefits and costs. Current and potential participants need to be "sold" on the personal benefits the program will provide them. In addition, promotional efforts need to be made frequently.

At the present time, there is no completed research available to substantiate the potential benefits that may be derived from employer-sponsored health and fitness programs. However, there is unanimous agreement among experts in the field that there are significant benefits derived from providing health and fitness programs to employees in a work place setting or for that matter to people associated with any other type of organization.

With reference to employee health promotion programs, Cohen writes:

> Such programs are proving beneficial to both employer and employee. Employee health programs have been shown to improve general health, reduce absenteeism and turnover, improve energy levels and reduce fatigue. Japan, which has the most advanced employee fitness programs, is also first in life expectancy and productivity. In short, good health is good for business.[66]

---

66. William S. Cohen, "Health Promotion in the Workplace," *American Psychologist.* 40:2, 214, February, 1985.

Shephard reports the following:

Possible sources of financial benefit from the development of a worksite exercise program (1) include an improved corporate image, facilitation of recruitment, an increase in the quality and quantity of production, decreased absenteeism, lesser turnover of employees, reduced health care costs and a lesser incidence of industrial injuries.[67]

He continues:

Against the various benefits of a worksite fitness program must beset the costs of facilities, equipment, leadership, opportunity and possibly an increased demand for some types of medical services.[68]

Managers, after reading what these two writers have to say about the benefits and costs of health and fitness programs, should have some basic information as to "selling" the program to top-level management and employees. They must keep in mind a very important point, however: health and fitness programs conducted at work sites benefit both the employer and the employee. It is absolutely essential that managers know how to "sell" the program to current and potential participants as well as to top-level management. After all, without participants there are no health and fitness programs.

At this point in the discussion it seems logical to define and discuss three terms that are closely linked: advertising, publicizing, and promoting.

Advertising is a paid form of nonpersonal communication about an organization, product, service, or idea by an identified sponsor.[69]

The key words that should be noted in the above definition are "paid," "non-personal," and "identified." The main purpose of advertising a health and fitness program is to "inform" or "persuade" people within an organization, a particular community, or geographic area to join the program. Obviously, paid advertising is not the way to promote the program within a work place, as the program can be publicized internally without paying for outside advertising.

Fallek offers the following list of the principal advertising media and the advantages and disadvantages of each:

---

67. Roy J. Shephard, "The Economic Benefits of Health and Fitness Programs," *Fitness in Business,* 2:3, 100, December, 1987.

68. Ibid., p. 102.

69. Eric N. Berkowitz, Roger A. Kerin and William Rudelius, *Marketing* (St. Louis, MO: Times Mirror/Mosby College Publishing, 1986), p. 431.

Newspaper

Advantages: High readership within geographic area; easy to reach metropolitan markets; frequent publication; short lead time; favorable for cooperative advertising; assistance available for copy and layout; volume and frequency discounts.

Disadvantages: Non-selective distribution within market; short life and brief exposure for any one ad; limited reproduction capability (poor quality of printing compared to magazines).

Magazine

Advantages: High degree of selectivity; long life; good to excellent reproduction quality; volume and frequency discounts; fairly thorough readership.

Disadvantages: Relatively high cost (which could be offset by results); long lead time.

Radio

Advantages: Good selectivity of audience through choice of station; can reach large audiences; flexible timing; short lead time; quick changes possible.

Disadvantages: Limited to audio; short life of message; subject to distractions while listening.

Television

Advantages: Very large audience possible; low cost per exposure; best communication impact via sight and sound; good selectivity of audience; high prestige.

Disadvantages: Highest production costs and high dollar costs for time; limited prime time available; short life of message; audience size not assured.

Direct Mail

Advantages: High selective as to type (letters, catalogs, price lists, brochures, circulars, newsletters, postcards, coupons, samplers, etc.); highest selectivity of audience; complete flexibility of timing; personal; stimulates action; hidden from competition; easy to measure.

Disadvantages: High cost of distribution; often discarded as "junk mail."

Outdoor

Advantages: Can be low cost; geographic selectivity; permits easy repetition; message "works" 24 hours a day.

Disadvantages: Brief exposure to public; message must be very short;

not selectivity of income level, age, education or other demographics other than geographic; considered by many to be a traffic hazard.[70]

Publicizing is "a nonpersonal, indirectly paid presentation of an organization, service or production. . . . [71]

The major difference between publicizing and advertising is the importance of the words "indirectly paid." When publicizing, indirectly paid takes into consideration the costs of the paper, postage, if appropriate, time to write or type a news release about a particular program, or time to call a reporter about a favorable newsworthy story about a program or a participant.

"Publicity has greater credibility than advertising."[72] Many readers consider an article about a particular health or fitness program or about a participant to be non-fiction.

Advertising has an axe to grind, but publicity is apparently objective news and features. Publicity benefits from an apparent "secondary endorsement" of it by the medium that chose to run it.[73]

In addition to a favorable news story, publicizing may also be in the form of an appropriate editorial or a particular program announcement. The following may help managers better to understand publicizing:

. . . A company can invite a news team to preview its innovative exercise equipment and hope for a favorable mention on the 6 p.m. newscasts. But without buying advertising time, there is no guarantee of any mention of the new equipment or that it will be aired when the target audience is watching. The company representative who calls the station and asks for a replay of the story may be told, "Sorry, it's only news once." With publicity there is little control over what is said, to whom, or when. . . . [74]

As for work places that conduct health or fitness programs or both, publicizing within organizations may include other forms such as pamphlets, booklets, brochures, catalogs, newsletters, flyers, fairs, conferences, bulletin boards, and word of mouth. The latter is one of the most effective methods of publicizing if a program(s) is of high quality. It is

---

70. Max Fallek, *How To Set Up Your Own Small Business*, Vol. 1 (Minneapolis, MN: American Institute of Small Business, 1987), (8) pp. 9–10.

71. Berkowitz, Kerin, and Rudelius, *Marketing*, p. 433.

72. Fallek, *Small Business*, (9) p. 5.

73. Ibid., (9) p. 5.

74. Berkowitz, Kerin and Rudelius, *Marketing*, p. 434.

surprising how fast the word gets around within an organization or within a community.

Managers should know the following guidelines for time, money and energy when publicizing: newspapers (50%), radio/television (25%), your catalog (10%), other publicity (15%).*

> Promoting "includes all the forms of communication (other than advertising) that call attention to the promotional idea or reinforce what is said in the advertising."[75]

For example, a manager of a community-based program will be introducing either a new health or a new fitness program and has already done a large amount of both advertising and promoting. Advertisements will be prepared for various kinds of media. Promoting the new health or new fitness program will entail having an evening during the week, Monday through Thursday, in which the manager will introduce the instructor who will make an oral presentation explaining the values and benefits of the program and, if a new fitness program is offered, will explain the use of the equipment. Of course, there will be time for a question-and-answer period at the end of the presentation. In addition, a flyer which will complement the oral presentation will be distributed to the audience and will indicate the cost of either the new health or the new fitness program.

Following are some ways for organizations to promote a health or fitness program for virtually little cost:

- *Free testimonials* — On each program's final evaluation, leave space for a short paragraph and a heading that reads: We would appreciate your comments to promote this program in the future.

_____

_____

_____

_____

Date   Signature, Address, Occupation

It is a good idea to use some of these endorsements when preparing the next brochure.

---

*Note: Percentages used are principally for community-based programs.

75. S. Watson Dunn and Arnold M. Barban, *Advertising, It's Role in Modern Marketing*, 6th ed., (New York, NY: The Dryden Press, 1986), p. 8.

- *Free mailing lists* — Exchange your lists for those held by other similar organizations. Perhaps the lists could be exchanged every three or four years. Although the other organization may not want yours, it may agree to exchange lists as a service, which could benefit both organizations.
- *Printing discounts* — Printers will sometimes give a discount in price if they are mentioned by name . . . "Printing by Acme."
- *Photos* — Take photographs of participants who are actually involved in this year's program to help promote next year's, if ongoing. Usually participants are pleased and flattered to have their pictures taken.
- *Free distribution of brochures* — Libraries, banks, school districts, state offices and other not-for-profit establishments are usually receptive to displaying these brochures.
- *Free media coverage* — There are many ways to get a story printed in magazines and newspapers and aired on radio and television. If the program is offered as not-for-profit, contact the public service director and ask how to prepare and submit the public service announcement.

The next section will provide managers with sound guidelines associated with public service announcements:

- Obtain a master list of all stations.
- Contact the key person, usually the public service director, learn his or her name and send all announcements to that individual.
- Be aware that radio and television spots run for 20 to 30 seconds but that announcements for newspapers may be longer.
- Keep sentences short, clear and well-written.
- Remember that radio stations need a minimum of ten days lead-up.
- Always include basic elements of who, what, where, when, and how.
- Double-space all announcements
- Try to space all announcements among different stations.
- Make sure to send thank-you's, whenever appropriate.

SUMMARY

Essential to any health and fitness program are financing and marketing. Before determining fees for health and/or fitness programs, managers will need to answer a series of questions in a definitive manner. Because there are no set standards for determining health and/or fitness program(s) fees, managers will need to analyze carefully responses to all questions and then draw their conclusions.

It is not a good idea for managers to act alone when setting up a fee structure for health and/or fitness program(s). It is recommended that a committee composed of either full-time or part-time staff members and a secretary, if available, be organized.

Because funding is crucial to any health and/or fitness program, in most cases, finding other financial resources becomes a real necessity. Knowing and understanding marketing is a must when health and/or fitness program(s) are offered. In order for managers better to understand marketing, they need to determine who the target audience is, what price the participant pays for the health and/or fitness program, what the program involves, where the program is to be delivered, and how the program is to be promoted.

Finally, three terms, *advertising, publicizing* and *promoting,* which are closely linked, are defined and discussed. A list of principal advertising media and the advantages and disadvantages of each is discussed. Also included are guidelines for time, money, and energy involved in publicizing. The chapter concludes by presenting some ways to promote a health and/or fitness program for very little cost.

Chapter X

LEADING THE HEALTH AND FITNESS PROGRAM: MEDICAL AND LEGAL CONSIDERATIONS

INTRODUCTION

Wherever health and fitness programs are conducted, two major areas, medical and legal, need to be considered and analyzed by managers. Although managers have several other responsibilities, these two areas have a profound effect on the participants, the staff and the program(s).

As professionals, managers should be constantly monitoring participants and be cognizant of all medical and legal matters that have a direct relationship to participants regardless of whether or not these participants are pursuing health or fitness programs or both. If either full-time and part-time instructors are employed, they too should have a general working knowledge of both the medical and legal areas, although the full responsibility lies with the manager. Although managers cannot make a final decision without first seeking a professional's advice, situations may arise that require consulting with an authority. If medical concerns surface, managers should consult the in-house physician, if available, or an outside physician. If legal, they should consult the in-house attorney, if available, or an outside attorney.

Managers should see that a safe and clear instructional environment is always available regardless of where the program(s) is located. Furthermore, it is important for the instructional staff to report to the manager any medical condition(s) and any legal matter and/or limitations participants presently have that can affect their performance in any fitness program.

MEDICAL CONSIDERATIONS

Health Education Programs

What medical considerations should be given to potential participants who wish to enroll in a health education program? Nowhere in the literature can the answer to this question be found. However, through a telephone survey, a group of health and fitness managers who offer health education programs were asked this question. The majority contacted replied that there were no medical considerations for those who wish to enroll in these types of programs. Participants themselves decide whether or not they wish to improve their health or change their health habits. One manager answered that medical considerations depend on the type of program that is being offered. One respondent said, "We have a form that potential participants are required to fill out at the time of registration and this form is used for only one particular program." Another respondent said, "We have a form for potential participants to fill out at the beginning of the program, but again this form is used for only one particular program."

It is recommended, whenever possible, that informational forms for all health education programs be provided to potential participants to be filled out at the time of registration or at the beginning of a program. This personal information will be extremely valuable to health education instructors and can assist them in designing programs based on the information found on the forms. Furthermore, each potential participant must be notified that all information will be kept confidential.

Fitness Programs

Medical considerations given to potential participants who wish to enroll in a fitness program will differ markedly from those of a health education program. These differences will be taken up so that a comparison can be made between the two programs. Hopefully, being aware of these differences may prove beneficial to managers who are planning or are presently offering either health education or fitness programs or both.

For many potential participants who wish to enroll in a fitness program, the pre-fitness evaluation, screening, or interview prior to entering a program is done by a fitness instructor, testing technician, or fitness counselor, if the latter two are available, in a private office. "Age, health status, type of test, and exercise plan are factors which determine the depth of evaluation required and need for medical involvement."[76]

The main reasons for the pre-fitness evaluation, screening, or interview are to provide information about a particular type of fitness program, to determine the potential participant's goals and objectives, and to discuss the medical clearance form, medical problems, and special needs, if any. In addition, the instructor will discuss the potential participant's medical history in order to determine the existing level of fitness, to recommend the appropriate mode of activity upon completion of the fitness tests, and to discuss the safety and liability concerns.

The pre-entrance requirements for those who wish to start a fitness program will differ from organization to organization. Some organizations require only a medical clearance form and the potential participant's signature on an informed-consent form. Other organizations are more comprehensive and require a pre-fitness evaluation, screening or an interview prior to administering either the maximal exercise test (graded exercise test) or the submaximal exercise test. If the potential participant is 40 years of age or over, a physician must be present when he or she does the maximal exercise test. If the potential participant is under 40 years of age, he or she does the submaximal test without a physician present.

In general, exercise testing is done for one of the following reasons:

1. To aid in the diagnosis of coronary heart disease in asymptomatic or symptomatic individuals
2. To assess the safety of exercise prior to starting an exercise program
3. To assess the cardiopulmonary functional capacity of apparently healthy or diseased individuals
4. To follow the process of known coronary or pulmonary disease and
5. To assess the efficacy of various medical and surgical procedures including the effect of medications.[77]

The chart below provides managers with the recommended entrance requirements for apparently healthy participants who wish to enter or reenter aerobic programs.

According to the American College of Sports Medicine, there are three major categories of potential participants who may wish to enter an exercise program:

---

76. American College of Sports Medicine, *Guidelines For Exercise Testing and Prescription*, 3rd ed. (Philadelphia, PA: Lea and Febiger, 1986), p. 1.

77. Ibid., pp. 1–2.

1. Apparently healthy—those who are apparently healthy and have no major coronary risk factors.
2. Individuals at higher risk—those who have symptoms suggestive of possible coronary disease and/or at least one major coronary risk factor.
3. Individuals with disease—those with known cardiac, pulmonary, or metabolic disease.

Results of exercise testing may dictate reclassification of individuals prior to prescribing an exercise program.[78]

ENTRANCE REQUIREMENTS—AEROBIC PROGRAMS FOR APPARENTLY HEALTHY PARTICIPANTS

NEW ENTRANT	FIT EVAL	MED HISTORY	PHYSICIANS MED	SUB-MAXIMAL OR GRADED EXERCISE TEST
age 34 and under	yes	yes	no	sm
Male 35–39 yrs	yes	yes	yes	sm
Female 35–44 years				
Male 40 yrs and over	yes	yes	yes	gxt
Female 45 yrs + over				
REENTER AFTER LESS THAN 1 YR ABSENCE				
For all ages	no	yes	no (unless change in med status)	if completed earlier—no
REENTER AFTER 1–3 YRS ABSENCE				
34 yrs and under	no	yes	no (unless change in med history)	" " " " "
Male 35–39 yrs	no	yes	yes	" " " " "
Female 35–44 yrs				
Male 40 yrs and older	no	yes	yes	" " " " "
Female 45 yrs and older				
REENTER GREATER THAN 3 YRS ABSENCE:	TREAT AS A NEW PARTICIPANT			

Note: All medical histories and doctors' medicals *must* be reviewed by either INSTRUCTOR, TESTING TECHNICIAN or EXERCISE COUNSELOR before acceptance. Staff, referring physician, or the medical director may require *more* stringent entrance requirements if clinical history requires it.

---

78. American College of Sports Medicine, *op.cit.*, p. 2.

Procedures for Emergency Action

Whether or not managers are instructing fitness classes, it is of utmost importance that they know and understand emergency action procedures. In most cases managers are not involved with fitness instruction. However, it is their responsibility to see that all full-time and part-time fitness instructors are properly trained in emergency action procedures. Accordingly, the following procedures are recommended:

- Make the participant as comfortable as possible.
- If possible, determine the nature of the injury or accident and take appropriate action by administering either basic first aid or cardiopulmonary resuscitation.
- If a nurse is available, ask a participant to contact him or her immediately for help. If not available, request help from a participant.
- Activate the emergency medical system, if needed.
- Dismiss the class, if advisable, and maintain order.
- Fill out the emergency action report form in detail.
- Obtain signatures of witnesses to the injury or accident.
- Notify the manager as soon as possible and forward the emergency action form to him or her to be kept on file for the record.
- If necessary, assure that the manager notify the next of kin as soon as possible.

LEGAL CONSIDERATIONS*

Fitness Programs

The organizer of a health club or health spa and the manager and staff of a fitness program are in a similar position when their exposure to a lawsuit is considered. Whether the program is free or whether it entails a costly membership fee, it remains open to the general public; so all who come have the status of invited guests. Some states make a distinction between a business invitee, such as a patron in

---

*This section was written by Richard S. Emerson, Jr., Attorney at Law, Portland, Maine.

a retail store, and a person who merely enters upon private property; but these distinctions are largely blurred in contemporary law. Therefore, for the sake of this discussion, the same duty is owed to anyone who is not a trespasser upon property. This means that, as far as the duty owed, a participant at an exclusive health club with five participants is equal to the person who uses the free exercise facilities which are open to the public.

We shall examine the ways in which a lawsuit can arise and how the spa owner, manager, or staff can take steps to avoid lawsuits and liability. We have lumped owners, directors, and managers together; they shall all be referred to as "managers." In most cases, fault may be attributed to the manager and/or staff members. Who actually might be responsible for payment of a judgment arising from a lawsuit is an entirely different question that is dependent on legal principles which cannot be appropriately dealt with here.

The first principle is to understand how lawsuits arise so they can be avoided. Sometimes, a lawsuit cannot be avoided, because unforeseen accidents will happen; but if the proper precautions have been taken to avoid the suit, there is a greater likelihood the manager or staff will not become liable for the injuries sustained in the accident.

Finally, we will discuss the ways in which liability can be limited by contractual agreements between the manager and the participants entered into prior to any accident.

Facilities Liability

When a participant uses the facilities at a health spa or is in a fitness program, injuries can occur which have nothing whatsoever to do with fitness or exercise. If the participant slips on the torn carpet on the way through the front door and is injured, a lawsuit is possible. The manager is responsible for the entire facility used by the participant regardless of whether the use is directly connected to the participant's reason for being there or not.

The duty of the manager is to exercise reasonable care to discover dangerous conditions which patrons cannot be expected to protect themselves against.[79] The manager owes the patrons a facility which is in reasonably safe condition.[80] Reasonable care, or due care, as it is

---

79. *Adam Dante Corp. v. Sharpe,* 483 S.W.2d 452 (Texas 1972).

80. *Bertrand v. Palm Springs & European Health Spa, Inc.,* 480 P.2d 424 (Oregon 1970).

sometimes called, does not become meaningful until discussed in the context of a particular accident.

For instance, let us suppose a health spa participant slips on the wet floor beside a pool. What does reasonable care mean in this instance? We know that there is little hope of keeping the area beside a pool free from water. If there was nothing which could be done to prevent the slippery condition which caused the fall, it might be said the manager used due care. But what if there is an indoor-outdoor carpet available, at a reasonable price, which could be used to prevent the slippery condition? In this way the question of reasonable care becomes one based upon the individual facts of a given situation. It is not a legal question. If a lawsuit were to be brought based on the above slip and injury, a jury would be given all the available data on what happened and what could have been done to avoid the accident. Then, they would be asked to decide if the manager used reasonable care in that instance.

The manager is in the same position as the proprietor of a business. He or she must use common sense and knowledge to keep the premises safe with reasonable care. Even if the manager makes a good-faith attempt to keep the premises safe but overlooks a hazard, this will not avoid liability. The standard which is used, that of reasonable care, assumes reasonable care will avoid accidents.

Faulty Equipment and Inadequate Instruction

It is obvious the manager must attempt to purchase fitness equipment which has been tested and proven. The staff must know how to maintain and use the equipment and, in addition, the manager and/or staff must not allow participants to use the equipment without proper instruction or assistance.

If injury occurs because a participant did not know how to use equipment properly, the question arise as to whether the staff was negligent in instruction on the safe use of the equipment. Staff members have a duty to instruct all participants on the safe use of each individual piece of equipment, including the dangers of using the equipment in an over-stressful manner. In addition, staffers should not assume any particular class of participant is more knowledgeable than another in this area; and after instruction, the manager should observe use of the equipment to be certain the instruction has been effective.

In most cases, a manager does not manufacture equipment or have any business relationship with the equipment manufacturer. Yet, if an injury occurs because of faulty equipment, the manager should not assume this is the manufacturer's problem only. Chances are, if a lawsuit is brought, the manager will be included under the theory that the equipment was not maintained properly or that the manager is "strictly liable" for faulty equipment.[81] Even if the injured party sues only the manufacturer, it is likely the manufacturer will [cross] complain against the staff member for failing to use, and the manager for failing to maintain, the equipment properly.

If equipment fails and causes an injury and a lawsuit, it will be a complex process of sorting out who is at fault. The important thing for the managers to remember is that their duty is to buy safe equipment and keep it in good working condition. Staff members need to prevent participants from hurting themselves because they do not know how to use the equipment safely.

Medical Injuries

Although the fitness facility is designed to improve health, occasionally the stress of exercise causes a sudden emergency. In order to determine what the duty of a manager is to avoid this sort of thing, we must divide the category of manager as we have not done before.

If a health spa opens its doors to the general public and provides a facility for its participants to exercise at will, without any particular program, the manager may assume participants will stress themselves to different degrees. Generally, it would be reasonable for the manager to limit the use of the facilities to participants who have been medically examined for weaknesses and ailments which might be aggravated by stressful exercise.

The situation becomes more complex when special exercise programs are involved. Then, the manager may be wise to consult with medical experts who can identify groups who might be at risk if involved in such a program. The manager should require a medical examination and health certification which is in accord with the special risks posed by the stresses of the particular program.

The highest duty to prevent medical emergencies exists in programs designed specifically as therapy for prior medical ailments or injuries. In these programs, the staff member is acting as a physical therapist who

---

81. *Marie v. European Health Spas, Inc.*, 434 NYS2d 802 (N.Y.A. pp. 1980).

knows the participants are there for treatment and have previously suffered from physical infirmity.[82]

Thus far, we have considered medical emergencies where there is a cause-and-effect relationship between stressful exercise and pre-existing weaknesses. There still remains the unforeseen emergency which cannot be medically predicted.

In one case[83] a participant at a health club went for a swim in the pool after a period of fairly stressful exercise. The participant suffered a medical emergency which nearly resulted in drowning. While the participant survived, there was permanent brain damage as a result. The spa was sued on a number of theories. These included the failure to provide a lifeguard, failure to determine the participant's physical impairments, failure to provide supervisory personnel, failure to warn of potential hazards, and failure to develop a detailed exercise program. The reported case decided only that the matter should be submitted to a jury where all the relevant circumstances could be established. This brings back the point that what is reasonable due care, even in the case of an unusual medical emergency, is a question decided by examining a myriad of factors surrounding the accident.

The manager is well advised to require medical certification to the degree that it assures a particular participant is fit for the program. The duty to avoid medical emergencies does not end with this certification, however, and other precautions may be necessary to handle the emergency if one does occur.

Contractual Agreements

It is not unusual for the health and fitness manager to ask its participants to sign an agreement specifying the nature of the facilities to be provided and the obligations of the participants as to payment of membership fees. These agreements may contain clauses designed to limit the liability of the health club. The participant may waive the right to sue the club for injuries arising during the course of activity at the club, and the participant may even agree to indemnify the owner of the club for injuries to third parties.

Any agreement is subject to a court test for validity when the occasion arises. Generally, courts have held that agreements limiting the lia-

---

82. *Bertrand v. Palm Springs & European Health Spa, Inc., supra.*

83. *Ely v. Northumberland General Ins. Co.,* 378 So.2d 1024 (Louis. 1979).

bility of health spas are enforceable if they are unambiguous in language and are clearly evident within the contract, rather than hidden in the middle of small print where the participant will not realize what is being agreed to.[84]

Another qualification on agreements is the special relationship which may exist between the parties (participant, staff and manager). If the participant was the voluntary participant of a private gym for recreational exercise, it is probable a waiver agreement would be valid.[85] The same agreement, between a participant recovering from a serious injury and the manager of a physical therapy program, might be invalid. In the second instance, the participant does not have the same freedom to refuse to sign the waiver as does the first participant. The physical therapy is needed for recovery from an injury, and it may be difficult or impossible for the person needing therapy to find another place where no waiver is required.

In any event, a waiver agreement can never limit liability for willful, wanton, or grossly negligent behavior. This means that an otherwise valid waiver does not allow a staff member and manager to ignore the duty of reasonable care and escape liability for an injury resulting from outright lack of care. In practical terms, this implies a waiver agreement limits the liability of a staffer and manager who has not been grossly negligent, but who accidentally overlooked a situation which caused harm to a participant. This makes sense in social policy terms. Were it otherwise, negligence would be encouraged.

Warnings

We all have seen the sign in the supermarket which says "caution wet floor." The warning sign can be used in certain instances to limit liability. Warnings can be used where dangers are discovered and it will take some time to correct the situation. Where certain activities or facilities are hazardous and there is no reasonable way to eliminate the hazard, a warning is appropriate.

The use of a warning has definite limits. It is not a liability waiver agreement. Warnings cannot take the place of due care, and, perhaps most important, they are not sufficient when people cannot be expected to heed the warnings and protect themselves. Thus, the "caution wet

---

84. See, for instance, *Empress Health & Beauty Spa, Inc. v. Turner*, 505 S.W.2d 188 (Tenn. 1973).

85. *Ciofalo v. Vic Tanney Gyms, Inc.*, 117 N.E.2d 925 (NY 1961).

floor" sign is fine when patrons can walk around the area, but if they must pass over the danger zone to get out the door, then the floor had better not be so slippery as to result in an injury.

One thing the warning does have in common with the waiver agreement is that it should always be conspicuous when used. The warning in small print on the wall under the towel rack which says the hot tub temperature is normally 112 degrees Fahrenheit may not be expected to prevent serious injury to the unwary participant.

Conclusion

There is no way to avoid positively the consequences of all accidents. Health and fitness managers can limit liability by taking reasonable steps to avoid injuries to participants and by entering into agreements to limit liability if and when there is an accident.

The individual, organization or manager responsible for a fitness program or spa should always seek the advice of an attorney who can analyze the particular problems faced in each instance. As we have indicated, no two situations are alike; and the approach to limiting liability which is suited to one organization may be inappropriate for another. The advice contained in this section is only intended to heighten the awareness of readers in the area of fitness program legal considerations. Because each program is structured differently to deliver certain benefits, the attorney working with the manager and staff can advise as to the specific considerations in each unique situation.

The safety expert is another good way to ferret out hazards the untrained eye may not detect. It may also be a safety expert who testifies, in court, as to the standard of care. It would do well to have the advice of an expert to rely on before a problem arises.

Keep in mind that the concept of reasonable care in negligence law is not static but may change with time as new methods are employed to assure the safety of participants on an "industry" wide basis. Another way of defining reasonable care is to observe what ordinarily passes for due care in similar situations. Each time an unanticipated event reveals a previously unknown hazard, the corrective steps taken as a result modify the status quo of the standard of care, and liability may depend upon staying abreast of the changing scene.

SUMMARY

Managers should be constantly monitoring participants and be cognizant of all medical and legal matters having a direct relationship to the participants. Full-time and/or part-time instructors should also have a general working knowledge of both the medical and legal areas.

Information forms filled out at the time of registration or at the beginning of the program will provide extremely helpful information to health education instructors and will also assist in the designing of programs.

For potential participants who wish to enroll in a fitness program, the pre-fitness evaluation, screening or interview prior to entering the program is required. Whether or not managers are instructing fitness classes, they must know and understand emergency action procedures, as they are totally responsible for the proper training of full-time and/or part-time instructors in emergency action procedures.

Managers and their staffs need to familiarize themselves with the steps to take in avoiding lawsuits and liability. Managers are entirely responsible in case of injury. It is the duty of the manager to exercise care to discover dangerous conditions which could cause an injury, such as faulty equipment or inadequate instruction.

There may be times when stress of exercise causes a sudden emergency. Therefore, generally, it would be reasonable for the manager to limit the use of the fitness facility to participants who have been medically examined for weaknesses and ailments which might be aggravated by stressful exercise.

All managers should have their participants sign an agreement form specifying the nature of the facilities to be provided, obligation as to payment of membership fees, and liability. However, any agreement is subject to a court test for validity if the occasion arises.

A warning sign may be used in certain instances to limit liability. Where certain activities or facilities are hazardous and there is no reasonable way to eliminate the hazard, a warning is appropriate.

Health and fitness managers can limit liability by taking reasonable steps to avoid injuries to participants and by entering into agreements to limit liability if and when there is an accident. It is the prudent manager who always seeks the advice of an attorney who can analyze the particular problems faced in each instance.

PART V
CONTROLLING THE HEALTH
AND FITNESS PROGRAM

Chapter XI

CONTROLLING AND EVALUATING THE HEALTH AND FITNESS PROGRAM

INTRODUCTION

I f a health and fitness program is to be top quality, it must be controlled and evaluated; both controlling and evaluating are ongoing processes. Managers should understand that these two areas have a significant impact on the program. Without adequate control and evaluation, no health and fitness program can achieve success.

Control and evaluation must also include the participants and staff. These two functions are interrelated with other managerial responsibilities and must receive a significant amount of attention. Therefore, in order for managerial control to be effective, standards should be established that determine what it is that needs to be controlled. First, health and fitness managers should gather information to find out if, in fact, there are any deviations from the established standards so that they can then take corrective action whenever and wherever there are any variations from the set standards.

Managers should also be cognizant of the fact that in order for evaluations to be effective they must have validity, reliability and objectivity. Obviously, evaluations are conducted to point out weaknesses. When these are discovered, action steps must be taken. Whenever evaluations are conducted and specific weaknesses are detected, unless fast corrective measures are taken, valuable time and financial resources will be wasted.

MEANING AND IMPORTANCE OF CONTROL

Managers of health and fitness programs may or may not be familiar with the word "control." This word, if not used in the proper context, can have negative overtones. For example, to some people the word control may mean powerful, autocratic, dictatorial, coercing, or domineering. Although these meanings may be correct when used in the appropriate context, control plays a necessary role in management. Silver provides the following definition of control as used in the field of management: "Control is the realizing or redirecting of efforts within predetermined standards to assure that planned goals are reached."[86] Simply stated with reference to health and fitness programs, control means keeping the program on course. Furthermore, in its essence, controlling also means monitoring the program closely in order to determine whether or not suitable progress is being made according to the established plan.

The importance of controlling as a health and fitness program managerial function has not really been accentuated because of the newness of health and fitness programs in such a variety of settings. However, controlling is utilized as a management function in various settings and has been used as such for many years.

Boone and Kurtz point out that accountability, rapidity of change, complexity and people's mistakes are factors that make controlling essential in today's organizations.[87] These four factors will be briefly explained as they relate to control within a health and fitness program.

Accountability

No one can deny that managers should be held accountable for health and fitness programs. In all cases, managers are accountable to their immediate supervisors, be it department heads, employee assistance program heads, or executive directors.

In order to be accountable, managers must know specifically what all their responsibilities are, how they themselves are to be evaluated, and what criteria are to be used in the evaluation. Accountability is almost impossible unless there is a controlling mechanism. Furthermore, since in large programs, managers may decide to delegate some of their responsibilities to a coordinator or a staff member, problems are bound to surface without an accountable control mechanism in place.

---

86. Gerald A. Silver, *Introduction to Management* (St. Paul, MN: West Publishing Co., 1981), p. 410.

87. Louis E. Boone and David L. Kurtz, *Principles of Management*, 2nd ed. (New York, NY: Random House Business Division, 1984), p. 411.

Rapidity of Change

In contemporary times, there are many rapid changes taking place in areas such as law, social values, technology, sports, and environment, resulting in many changes within the health and fitness fields. All one has to do is to examine and compare health education programs and fitness programs that were conducted in the 1970s with those of the 1980s. How fast these programs are changing! Because changes are occurring so rapidly in health and fitness programs, ongoing evaluation and reevaluation of the goals and objectives of these programs are urgent. Therefore, a controlling mechanism must be established to discover changes that have an impact on these programs.

Complexity

Health and fitness programs are complex, as both these areas are deep-rooted in science. As health and fitness programs grow by an increasing number of participants and by the addition of new programs, a controlling mechanism is required. With growth, decentralization usually occurs, necessitating additional staff. Consequently, methods for controlling the staff must be implemented.

People Mistakes

Staff members, like all other human beings, make mistakes. Unlike computers, a staff person cannot be programmed to perform specific duties. Health and fitness managers cannot consistently predict how accurately a staff member will respond to instruction, authority, and leadership. An effective controlling mechanism should be able to identify mistakes made by staff members and then take action to correct these mistakes as soon as possible.

THE CONTROL PROCESS

"There are three distinct stages in the control process. These are setting standards, comparing performance to standards and taking necessary corrective action. . . ."[88]

---

88. Mescon, Albert, and Khedouri, *Management,* p. 383.

Setting Standards

A good definition of standards that seems appropriate for this book is the following. Standards are "something established for use as a rule or basis of comparison in measuring or judging capacity, quantity, content, extent, value, quality, etc."[89]

The control process is another of the health and fitness manager's responsibilities; but, when appropriate, the staff should be involved. Standards are the derivative of the planning process and serve as reference points for comparing performance. Furthermore, these standards are closely related to the goals of a health and fitness program. Therefore, it is absolutely essential that when planning takes place, standards should be established. Moreover, it is important that all standards be derived from the goals and planning strategies of the health and fitness programs. Managers of health and fitness programs should become familiar with three types of standards: standards of instruction, standards of professional ethics and responsibility, and standards of participant achievement. "Standards of instruction" refers to methods and techniques used in teaching health education and fitness programs. Also involved is establishing a good instructor/participant relationship. "Standards of professional ethics and responsibility" are concerned with the ideals of the profession. Moreover, they involve participation in professional associations. And "standards of participant achievement" refers to testing participants in health education and fitness or both so as to determine the amount of progress.

Comparing Performance to Standards

Standards of instruction can be readily evaluated by observation, written and/or oral reports and consultation with staff members. Teaching performance can be evaluated in a relatively short time. Also, standards of professional ethics and responsibility of staff members are quickly discovered. Being an active member of a professional organization is usually an indication of professionalism.

With respect to standards of participant achievement, whenever possible, a comparison of performance should be made to standardized or instructor-prepared tests in health education and to tests of submaximal or maxi-

---

89. Guralnik, *Webster's*, p. 1387.

mal fitness. Participants may also compare their previous performance with their present performance over a specified period of time. In some cases, level of achievement may be compared to that of other members of the class.

Taking Necessary Corrective Actions

Once standards have been implemented and after an appropriate period of time has passed, managers must decide upon which one of the three courses of action is to be taken. "The three courses of action are to do nothing, to correct the deviations, or to revise the standards."[90]

Do Nothing

The major purpose of control is to determine whether or not the management process is proceeding in accordance with the standards or plan. There may be cases when everything is going well. When a comparison of results to standards indicate that the standards are being attained, the best course of action is to do nothing. However, health and fitness managers cannot assume that when everything is going well during a certain period of time, they will remain the same way during some other period of time. Keep in mind that managers change and so do standards. However, if the control process indicates that everything is going according to the standards, all the manager needs to do is to measure performance again, thus repeating the control cycle.

Correct Deviations

Obviously, there may be times when there are deviations from the established standards. When deviations occur, managers need to know exactly what and where they are and what needs to be done to correct them. What action health and fitness managers take to correct these deviations depends upon their analysis of these mistakes. In most cases, in health and fitness programs, the manager's major concerns are environmental factors, qualifications of staff members, motivation, and dismissals.

---

90. Mescon, Albert, and Khedouri, *Management*, p. 389.

Environmental Factors

Facilities and equipment availability, class size, and classifications of participants are the major physical concerns of health and fitness managers that can impede instructors from reaching the established standards. Inadequate facilities and unsatisfactory equipment, large classes, and classifying participants particularly in fitness programs are hindrances facing instructors.

Some of the above factors can be more readily rectified than others. From the standpoint of cost, the most expensive item are facilities. However, without a substantial amount of money it would be impossible to build a facility or additional facilities.

Qualification of Staff Members

In some cases, when staff members fail to attain established standards, the question arises as to what corrective action should be taken. Accordingly, two possible ways to eliminate a staff member's incompetence is to recommend that he or she attend institutes, conferences, seminars, and workshops and/or take professional academic courses in his or her speciality area. In addition, managers may initiate in-service training programs.

Motivation

Often, staff members are not performing up to expectations. Staffers cannot reach their established standards unless they are properly motivated. The duty of all managers should be to have all staff members reach their maximum performance. (An in-depth discussion on motivating the staff for performance may be found in Chapter VIII.)

Dismissals

As a last resort, managers may dismiss or terminate a staff member. Obviously, dismissals are always involuntary and permanent. Although dismissals occur infrequently, managers are sometimes forced to take this action. Once all other avenues have been exhausted and a staff member has not even attempted to improve his or her performance, the end result has to be dismissal. But before dismissing a staff member, managers need to make a strong case for the termination. Also, if employees are in a union, this union will want a full account as to the reasons for the dismissal.

INSTRUMENTS OF CONTROL

Although there are a variety of instruments of control available to health and fitness managers, the seven major ones are as follows:

Policies and Procedures

One of the most effective of all control techniques is the utilization of the policies and procedures by all full-time and part-time staff. These represent the most suitable ways by which staff members can perform their duties, and managers can use control through such policies and procedures. When managers see to it that staff members adhere to and use all the policies and procedures, the program(s) are bound to be of high quality.*

Programs

The key to any comprehensive health and fitness program are the programs or components that are currently being offered and those that are planned for implementation in the future. Therefore, controlling the programs becomes crucial. What actually needs to be controlled are the quality, number, and variety of programs that are to be conducted. Of course, the variety must be predicated on need. Monitoring all programs is also a part of this controlling tool.

Schedules

Managers need to give a good amount of time to the scheduling of health education and fitness classes. Although time consuming, it is an important control technique. In some organizations, the scheduling of classes must coincide with the employee work schedules.

Staff and Instruction

Staff members are not given the freedom to instruct in whatever program they wish. They are assigned by the manager to teach in a particular program. There may be a staff member who likes diversifica-

---

*An in-depth discussion on policies and procedure may be found in Chapter V.

tion and may request a change of an instructional assignment, for example, from teaching the smoking-cessation program to teaching the stress management program or from teaching the walk/jog program to teaching weight training.

Participants and Classes

With respect to control, participants, staff and programs are interrelated. Health education participants can be controlled by the following three techniques: limiting the class size, setting a specific time allotment for each class session, and determining the number of classes participants must attend in order to complete a program. Fitness participants can be controlled by limiting the class size, having a specific time allotment for each class session, setting age limits, determining test norms or criteria for passing the fitness test, and setting the number of classes participants must attend in order to complete a program.

Facilities*

If an organization has its own facilities, these are always controlled by the manager. The scheduling of these facilities is the only control technique used. If a conference or meeting room is available, it is scheduled for health education classes. If a gymnasium or multi-purpose room is available, it is scheduled for fitness classes. Of course, the maintenance and cleanliness of the facility are also the manager's responsibility.

Budgets

No one can argue that the budget is the most powerful instrument of control. Many of the goals managers want to achieve fail because funds are not available.

Managers can employ financial resources to control many of the components and activities within the comprehensive health and fitness programs. (An in-depth discussion on budgets follows.)

---

*An in-depth discussion on facilities may be found in Chapter VII.

BUDGETS*

Budgets were briefly discussed above as a control instrument, but the word was never defined; therefore, it seems appropriate that it be defined in this section.

"A detailed financial plan often including detailed income, work and resource allocation plans for carrying out a program of activities in a specific time period, often a fiscal year,"[91] is called a budget.

The purpose of the budget process is to determine the distribution of resources from one organizational unit or function to another, for example, from a university or business to a department, from a department to a health and fitness program, from the program to the various program components. In determining budget allocations, explicit choices are made among alternative ways in which resources might be used. The central question becomes, then, On what basis should it be decided to allocate X dollars to activity A rather than activity B?

The budget has two additional functions. It is an instrument for translating priorities and plans into actions. In a purely rational world, a set of priorities would establish the relative importance of various institutional goals for the coming budget period and resources would then be allocated to activities according to those priorities. The budget also serves as an instrument for achieving both internal and external accountability. It is a mechanism for expenditure and management control of operational programs and for communicating to constituencies the activities that will be supported by allocations and the expected results. Historically, the emphasis in budgeting in public organizations has been more on control than on program planning and evaluation, though that balance has shifted somewhat in recent years.

A budget for an organization, a unit or a program is a document that combines a statement of activities for a given period of time with information about the funds required to engage in those activities or to achieve the programmatic objectives of those activities. For the health and fitness manager, the two most direct concerns about budgeting are, first, how

---

*This section was written by Doctor Robert J. Goettel, Executive Assistant to the President, University of Southern Maine, Portland, Maine, and portions were adapted from T Husen and T N Postlethwaite, eds., *The International Encyclopedia of Education*, Vol. 1 (Pergamon, Oxford: Pergamon Press Ltd., 1985), pp. 585–588.

91. Daniel Oran and Jay M. Shafritz, *The MBA's Dictionary* (Reston, VA, Reston Publishing Company, Inc., 1983), p. 58.

through the budget process can I obtain the necessary resources to realize the goals of my program? And second, how can I use the process of budget development and management to make the very best use of those resources that are made available to my program?

One view treats the process of developing and administering budgets simply as a technical exercise used by managers to control organizational activities and to assure accountability. But when the process is seen instead as a major policymaking tool, budget development and administration become a politically dynamic rather than simply a technical endeavor. In most organizations, budgets and budget development are instruments of both accountability and policy planning. The particular form of a budget and an organization's approach to the budget development process will reflect the primary purpose.

Types of Budgets

Budget types can be described as (1) line item, (2) performance, or (3) program.

Line-Item Budget

The line-item budget presents expenditures by type of object, i.e., salaries, supplies, equipment, and travel. This type of budget provides a high degree of control over what an organization spends its resources on. Some organizations limit the extent to which the budget manager has the authority to shift funds from one budget category to another (say, supplies to travel) without approval of superiors or the governing board. Line-item budgeting can be combined with performance or program budgeting.

Performance Budget

A performance budget is useful for planning and evaluation purposes if the major focus is on the level of productivity or work loads required to carry out a program or components. In a health and fitness program, such activities might include fitness testing, in-service training, and services. This can be a useful way to construct a budget when the level of program expenditures is primarily a function of unit costs times the number of participants.

Program Budget

Within a large organization, the health and fitness program may well have a single budget. But the manager also may wish to know more about individual components of his or her area that relate directly to program objectives; for example, nutrition and weight management, smoking cessation, aerobic dance, and weight training.

Traditional Approaches to Budget Development

For the manager, the principal budget question is, How much did you get compared to (1) what your unit received last year and (2) competing units or programs? This means that you must understand both the techniques and the politics involved in the process of determining organizational budget levels.

Most public organizations use one or a combination of the following five approaches to developing budgets and determining allocations to organizational units.

Incremental Budgeting

Under this, the most common form of budgeting, incremental increases are permitted in each line item of the organization or program's budget. The main assumption behind the incremental budgeting is that the existing basis for allocating resources is appropriate and that present programs are to be continued in their current form. The strength of this approach is its stability and predictability; its weakness is the limited extent to which units or programs are encouraged to justify existing expenditures that may not be productive. Health and fitness managers with limited resources and creative ideas will be constrained in their ability to disproportionately expand their budgets under an incremental approach.

Open-Ended Budgeting

This approach calls for the health and fitness program along with all other units to submit a budget request at the level considered by the unit appropriate to meet program needs. Usually through a process of negotiation, the unit head and central budget officials adjust the budget to match available resources. Increased opportunity for unit program planning and participation is balanced by the frequent incompatibility of requests and available resources and the absence of clear criteria for reaching final allocation decisions. Powerful and influential unit heads with strong constituencies tend to experience greater success under this approach.

Quota Budgeting

Sometimes referred to as a lump-sum budget, this approach is directly opposite to open-ended budgeting. Institutional cost centers are given a control figure and then requested to build a line-item budget based on this allotment. Decentralization of budget authority over line items which can encourage flexibility and effective unit planning is balanced by central administration's reliance on previous budget amounts and a uniform treatment of all program areas.

Alternative-Level Budgeting

Several budget levels are presented in this approach, that is, 10 percent below current, 5 percent below, 5 percent above. By forcing unit managers to prepare alternate levels, central administration can obtain a rough classification of program priorities and details of program evaluations within units based on the judgments of managers of operating units. Like the approaches above, this one is largely a function of budget levels from prior years.

Formula or Revenue Budgeting

This approach focuses on quantitative measures of the current financial need of individual units where the measures of need or participation are the same across units. A variation on this approach ties the funds available to the revenue generated by each unit's program activities. The advantages are that this approach is seen as comparable to the way a business is operated, in that both entrepreneurial and cost-effective behavior is encouraged. The disadvantage is that resources allocated may not match either average or marginal unit costs of program operation. This will be a particular concern when the health and fitness program has little or nothing to say about how unit charges are determined.

Rational Approaches to Budgeting

By the late 1960s, governing boards of many public organizations and institutions sought more "business-like" and more accountable mechanisms for making "better" choices among competing program resource requests. The expectation was that more credible approaches would produce greater public support. Rational budgeting approaches were based on classical theories of economic efficiency. The intent was to reduce the influence over resource allocations of historical spending patterns and the political power of strong unit managers and constituencies. The two most commonly tried "rational" approaches have been Planning, Programming, and Budgeting (PPB), a highly centralized approach to budget decision making, and Zero-Based Budgeting (ZBB), which is more decentralized in character.

Planning, Programming and Budgeting

Traditional budgeting methods were seen as not output-oriented, focused more on the past than the future, not clearly identifying program choices, focused on resources rather than results, and not suggesting how resources were related to goals. PPBS, on the other hand, introduced into contemporary budgeting practice the more explicit consideration of objectives in making budget choices; the consideration of multi-year rather than single-year costs; the analysis of alternative means of accomplishing objectives; and an evaluation of the benefits or effectiveness of the budget choice. Planning involves the identification and selection of overall long-range organizational goals and the analysis of alternative ways of achieving those goals. Programming requires decisions on the specific course of action to be followed in implementing planning decisions. And budgeting involves translating those decisions into financial plans. The planning and programming components are directed by centralized budget authorities.

Zero-Based Budgeting

PPB is primarily concerned with broad policy decisions and centralized, top-down decision making. Zero-based budgeting is designed to transform objectives for individual program units into an efficient operating plan by total justification of every activity from base zero to build a new budget. Decision packages for each program objective are developed which describe the costs and benefits of alternative actions, work load and performance measures, and various levels of effort. The core of the ZBB approach is formalized comparisons of alternative expenditures.

While traditional approaches to budgeting have a number of weaknesses based on historical patterns of funding, the more rational approaches clearly have their limits as well. These include difficulties in measuring program outcomes, establishing clear relationships between program resources and outcomes, and accurately determining program costs. They also require a substantially greater use of staff, manager and central decision-maker time. Moreover, it is not at all clear that the use of rational budgeting approaches has resulted in significant reallocations of program resources.

The health and fitness manager can expect to encounter efforts at more rational budget decision making when program reductions are required. They may be most effective for service and support functions rather than core program activities. They certainly produce more awareness of program costs, particularly long-term costs, and they can focus attention on the implications, particularly long-term, of financial decisions.

Criteria for a Good Budget

A good budget development and management process accomplishes the following:

1. It reflects the programmatic priorities of the organization's governing board and executive leadership.
2. It provides a level of resources appropriate to realizing program goals and objectives.
3. It permits evaluation and analysis of the relationship between resource allocations and the attainment of organizational goals.
4. It provides appropriate control of expenditures consistent with budget allocation decisions.
5. It allows program managers and budget officers to identify and address unplanned financial emergencies.
6. It facilitates accountability for the use of resources on the part of the organization's administrators.

Preparation and Planning

Careful preparation for submitting a budget request requires (1) analysis of current expenditure patterns relative to program objectives, (2) careful consideration of expanded or new program initiatives, and (3) attention to the actors in and the dynamics of the budget process.

Analyzing Current Budget Performance

Careful management of current budget performance means that you have monitored and controlled expenditures to the best of your ability given expected program performance demands. Every budget experiences unexpected pressures: unplanned repairs or replacement of equipment, and additional program participants that require more staff resources. The first step in the preparation process is to explain discrepancies in previous and current year budget performance compared to expectations. Why did the discrepancies occur? Are the reasons that led to them likely to continue or were they single time events? What, if any, are the implications for future spending?

A related step concerns comparing budget performance against program performance. Were the components of your program implemented as intended? Were your program goals and objectives realized? If not, were the reasons related to budget performance? Would resources deployed differently correct the problem or are additional resources required? What, if any, are the budget implications of your new plans to achieve program objectives, or should those objectives be modified? Each program budget that you submit should be designed to achieve the objectives to which you and your supervisors have agreed.

Expanded or New Program Initiatives

Your evaluation of current budget performance may lead to expanded or new program initiatives, or such requests may result from an expansion of your assigned program goals and objectives. You will need to tie new budget requests to specific goals and objectives by analyzing the resource requirements of expanded or new programs.

The Budget Cycle

A health and fitness program budget cycle is usually annual. Most organizations therefore begin preparation of the following year's budget shortly after beginning implementation and management of the current budget. At the same time, the organization will be closing out and conducting an evaluation of the previous year's budget and expenditures. The health and fitness program manager will be preparing the budget proposal for the following year based on solid expenditure information that is two years' old, estimated information about the current year that is only partially complete, and the manager's estimates of the costs of new or expanded program initiatives. This places a special value on good information and on understanding of the program's expenditure patterns and cost structure. The better your knowledge of current patterns and problems, the more realistic and credible your proposal for funding in the following year. Many organizations present budget proposals that include data for all three years. Where line-item or subprogram increases are more than incremental, the program manager is expected to provide complete justification of those increases.

The Budget Game

The budget game in any large organization or agency is played by many actors in addition to you, your supervisor and the budget officer. They include other administrators such as yourself who are going through the same steps and competing for the same funds as you. Each of your competitors will try to make the strongest case possible for obtaining a disproportionate share of scarce resources.

They also include the chief executive officer of your organization. His or her responsibility is to balance competing requests in light of his or her and the governing board's goals and priorities for the organization and an assessment of relative needs.

The interest groups associated with the various program units in your organization represent an important set of actors in the budget decision-making process. You will need to analyze the relative presence and strength of interests supporting your program and competing programs and then determine how your support can best influence budget decisions. For the health and fitness manager, satisfied program participants can be an important source of program support. In doing so, you will need to be sensitive to potential negative reactions by chief executive officers and governing board members to pressure strategies seen as outside accepted approaches to influencing policy decisions.

Finally, governing board members are key actors in the budget decision-making process. Different members have different special interests in the organization and play different roles in the decision process. How you structure your case for additional funding should at least in part be based on a careful analysis of the board's current interests and priorities.

Managing Budget Performance

Once allocation decisions are made, an approved budget is established for the health and fitness program. The program manager is then responsible for budget management over the course of the fiscal year. Managerial accounting involves (1) collecting financial transaction data through a management information system, (2) generating reports which enable managers to control performance, and (3) auditing.

Transactional data are bits of information about pay rates, expenditures, and purchase orders routinely collected by accounting and payroll systems. *Control data* are developed by producing reports that compare budget categories of transaction data with budget performance expectations. Many organizations produce control reports for program managers that reflect only *expenditures,* a bill for an item or a service that has actually been paid. Some organizations are able to include in control reports *obligations,* an agreement to purchase an item or a contract to pay an employee or consultant. And some other organizations include commitments to current employees in addition to expenditures but do not include other obligations. The program manager is best served when the control report provides an accurate, up-to-date picture of uncommitted resources after all expenditures and obligations have been included.

A monthly financial report should show the program's expenditures (bills actually paid) for the month compared to budget, year-to-date expenditures and uncommitted funds. There may well be planned uses for the uncommitted funds; to date neither a contractual commitment nor a purchase order has been issued to formally limit the use of those funds. The assumptions behind the report's monthly and year-to-date data must be understood by the program manager. Rarely do program units or departments spend at the same rate each and every month. The program manager will need to know whether the report is based on an assumption of equal monthly spending or on projections of monthly variations in spending.

When expenditures and obligations covering a given period of time are properly recorded, it can be determined whether they have occurred for the purposes allowed by law and/or by the organization's financial policies. The process for making such determinations is called *auditing.* All public organizations are subject to periodic audits by both internal and external auditors for this purpose. A good financial management system will facilitate good accounting practices and reduce the possibility of audit exceptions.

In Conclusion

What is good budget development and management? How can the health and fitness manager use the process to obtain and make the best use of available resources? Here are some bromides for success.

1. *Live within your current budget.* Superiors and budget officers do not like cost overruns. Learn how to read expenditure reports. Stay on top of future spending. Make adjustments within your budget to compensate for expenditure patterns different from what was expected. Most important, remember that budget officials especially do not like surprises. If problems arise that cannot be handled within your current budget, raise the issue with your superior and the budget officer and develop a plan for addressing the problem.

2. *Understand your program's costs.* Learn what your program and its various components are actually costing. Identify those elements that you could control versus those that are uncontrollable. Know your program's budget better than your superiors and the budget official.

3. *Understand how your process of budget allocation and management works.* Learn what steps or actions are required and when. Submit reports and requests on time, with the correct forms properly completed. Learn what factors influence decisions about allocations to your program. Always do your homework.

4. *Be accurate and realistic in your budget proposals.* While most managers request more than they expect to receive, your requests must have accurate cost estimates and they must be plausible. The process of budget development provides superiors and budget officers one of the best indicators of whether your program is well managed. Budget officers always believe that they know which programs have slack resources that, given budget reductions, can be employed to achieve program goals.

5. *Connect budget requests to long-term program planning.* Rational strategies like PPB and ZBB are designed to promote long-range program planning and systematic examination of alternatives. Your budget

development and management strategies can be strengthened by bringing these perspectives to bear on traditional approaches even when the techniques of rational budgeting are not required.

6. *Generate demand for your program.* The best case for more resources is greater demand. Learn how to create participation and how to translate participants into a constituency to support your budget requests.

MEANING AND IMPORTANCE OF EVALUATION

The word "evaluation," as defined here, is a process of gathering and analyzing information whereby an estimation or judgment may be made as to the amount of value given. In those instances where goals are based on attainment of pure numeric data, evaluation is self-determined by the results. Goals of an intangible nature require a thorough review of the results and the application of individual judgment to determine the degree to which the goal was met or partially met.

Evaluation is the major responsibility of health and fitness managers. The need for evaluation is present in any contemporary, viable and dynamic program as well as in organizations. For only when outcomes are measured against original purposes or stated goals will managers be able to judge progress. With the proper amount of resources, managers are expected to accomplish the objectives for which their programs were started. The manager's goal is the highest level of accomplishment of his or her program's objectives. This goal requires the maximum contribution of all staff members. It is imperative that managers evaluate the achievements of their staffs individually and collectively to determine how successful they have been and how their work may be improved in the future. In addition, the program and participants need to be evaluated.

Some health and fitness managers contend that their many responsibilities leave no time to devote to evaluation. Evaluation is like bookkeeping in business; it indicates direction and reveals degrees of accomplishment. It is vital that all managers give a great deal of attention to evaluation, as failure to do so will result in less than effective managerial practices.

Program Evaluation

Rutman and Mowbray define program evaluation as "the use of scientific methods to measure the implementation and outcomes of programs, for decision-making purposes."[92] Program evaluation plans should include both formative and summative questions and procedures.

Formative Evaluation

Formative evaluation tells managers if their programs are on schedule and are being implemented as planned. More important, formative evaluation identifies those components of plans and resource-allocation decisions that must be modified to achieve goals and objectives. The following questions are asked regularly throughout the course of each program and/or fiscal year. Are we on target with respect to plans? If not, why not? What problems are occurring? What, if any, mid-course corrections should be made? Should the budget be changed and resources redeployed? What modifications should be made in future activities based on current experiences and findings? Many organizations conduct formal mid-year budget reviews which address these questions. The process is especially important for those health and fitness programs dependent on fee income to support program activities.

Summative Evaluation

A summative evaluation determines whether program goals have been achieved over the course of the entire program. Summative evaluation procedures are closely tied to the process of long-term or strategic planning for an ongoing program. The types of questions asked include: Has the program been a success? If not, why not? What are the implications of those answers for the design of continuing program activities and for the program's overall mission? Should specific areas of program focus be continued and in what form? What are the implications for budget development? Perhaps the most important concern for the health and fitness program manager is to reach agreement with participants, superiors and governing boards about how the program will be judged and what specific indicators will be used to measure success. Conflict and frustration are the typical by-products of an organizational environment

92. Leonard Rutman and George Mowbray, *Understanding Program Evaluation* (Beverly Hills, CA: Sage Publications, 1983), p. 12.

where the expectations of key stakeholders and decision makers differ from those of the program manager.

Staff Evaluation

Performance evaluation is the periodic appraisal of a staff member's job performance measured against the position's stated or presumed requirements.[93] The manner in which a health and fitness staff member performs his or her job in terms of quantity and quality will determine to a great extent the success of the program.

The need for performance evaluation of a staff cannot be over-emphasized. Performance evaluation of a health and fitness staff is the responsibility of the manager. However, receiving feedback, a form of evaluation, from coworkers is also valuable as an aid in improving a staff member's performance.

Prior to the performance evaluation, managers should prepare themselves by reviewing the following suggestions:

Suggestions For Health Education Instructor Evaluation Areas
Class Organization and Content

Are the objectives of the program clearly defined?

Are the classes organized?

Are the content areas prepared in advance?

Are the lectures given at the proper level so as to be understandable?

Are educational media materials and the necessary hardware an integral part of the lectures?

Are the health needs, interests and problems of the participants considered?

Does the instructor provide answers to questions asked by participants?

Is there follow-up on questions asked by participants?

Does the instructor have, or is he or she making a reasonable effort to acquire knowledge in the health education field?

Is the instructor confident in his or her knowledge of the program?

---

93. Adapted from Terry and Franklin, *Principles*, p. 386.

Personal/Interpersonal Contact

Is the instructor available for a few minutes after each class for discussion with participants?

Is the instructor enthusiastic about the program?

Is the instructor concerned about the quality of his or her teaching?

Is the instructor proficient in providing feedback to participants?

Are the instructor's personal appearance and mental attitude consistent with that of a proper role model?

Suggestions for Fitness Instructor Evaluation Areas Class Organization and Content

Are directions and announcements given clearly?

Are exercise durations according to protocol?

Are all participants given proper levels of exercise?

Are remedial exercises given when necessary?

Are routines varied and pace changes given to sustain interest levels?

Are exercises/dances explained and demonstrated properly?

Does the instructor have, or is he or she making a reasonable effort to acquire a working knowledge of the fitness field?

Are educational needs of beginners met via discussions of oxygen, recovery rates, exercise, heat, and so forth?

Does the instructor provide answers to questions asked by participants?

Is follow-up done on questions, including those concerning injury to a participant?

Is the instructor observant during class?

Personal/Interpersonal Contact

Is the instructor available a few minutes before and after class for consultation with participants?

Is the instructor enthusiastic?

Is the instructor accessible to participants? Do participants feel comfortable in approaching the instructor for advice or discussion?

Is the instructor proficient in providing feedback and reinforcement to participants?

Are the instructor's personal appearance, exercise level, and life-style consistent with that of a proper role model?

Participant Evaluation

Health Education

The best way to evaluate the knowledge of a potential participant about a particular health education program is to administer a pre-test. Upon completion of the program, the same test is administered as a post-test. Comparison of the pre-test scores with those of the post-test will, of course, indicate what the participant has learned by taking the program.

Some health education tests are standardized, while others are instructor-prepared. In both types of tests, the instructor is seeking either general or specific health information. These tests may be of various types, for example, true or false, multiple choice, or essay.

Fitness

No one can argue that fitness evaluations are completely different from health education evaluations. The former centers on knowledge attained after completion of a particular health education program(s). The latter focuses on the participant's present fitness level and the progress he or she has made toward reaching a satisfactory level upon completion of a program(s). They, too, may wish to be post-tested. Fitness evaluations include specific areas, namely, height, weight, body fat composition, postural strength, upper and lower maximal body strength, pulmonary function, cardiovascular or aerobic capacity, and flexibility. As a conclusion to this section, fitness evaluation goals are listed:

- To establish a baseline fitness level
- To provide incentives for improvement
- To establish performance goals
- To provide a basis of comparison for re-evaluation
- To write an exercise prescription.

USING FITNESS DATA*

Described here are types of analyses that could be performed on physical measurements such as weight, blood pressure, bench press, leg

---

*This section was written by Paul Rogers, Professor of Mathematics and Statistics, University of Southern Maine, Portland, Maine.

press, flexibility, oxygen intake, etc. Measurements could be taken on a continuing basis as new participants enter a fitness program with follow-ups as desired. Each participant could be categorized by sex, age, weight class, or by any other categorical variable of interest.

Variables such as weight and age can be categorized by establishing groups. For example, managers could have:

> AGE CLASS 1:   Ages between 20 and 29
> AGE CLASS 2:   Ages between 30 and 39,
> etc.

What can health and fitness managers do with the data collected? Here are two examples of what can be done:

1. Managers can establish norms for the physical variable for the various classes of participants in the program. This can be done by finding the mean and standard deviation for the physical measurement for those participants in each category of interest. Managers can, for example, find the means and standard deviations of oxygen intake for females by weight class and age class. If there were seven weight classes and six age classes, one would have forty-two sets of norms. The norms obtained will be useful only if the number of observations in each of the forty-two groups is reasonably large. If the manager wants to use a measure of variation other than the standard deviation, he or she can use the interquartile range. One can also use percentiles to indicate how the measurement is distributed.

2. Managers can look for relationships between the variables. This can be accomplished by:

   a. Using contingency tables (chi-square) techniques or using log-linear models.

   b. Using regression techniques to see if there is an equation which relates a "response variable" with one or more "explanatory variables." One can, for example, search for a relationship between flexibility (the response variable) and weight, age, and oxygen intake. This type of analysis might shed some light on how much a measurement changes when other variables change.

Indicated are only a few of the possibilities available to the manager who wants to explore the measurements associated with fitness programs. The analysis is predicated upon using computing facilities, either a mainframe computer or micro computer with the appropriate statistical software. Software packages which will perform almost any desired analysis are SAS (mainframe or micro), SPSS (mainframe or micro), Systat (micro, PC or Mac.), and BMD (mainframe or micro).

Much can be learned from a data set by using simple statistical methods such as computing means and quartiles, and making histograms, stem-leaf plots, box plots, and scatterplots. Getting familiar with the data by using these elementary tools will prompt further, perhaps more sophisticated, inquiry which may require the services of a statistical consultant.

SUMMARY

Control is central to health and fitness programs; for without it, managers will be unable to keep the programs on course. Furthermore, control monitors the program closely in order to determine whether or not satisfactory progress is being made according to the established plan.

Controlling a health and fitness program is an important function that has really not been accentuated, perhaps because of the newness of the health and fitness programs and the failure to realize that control is one of the responsibilities of managerial positions.

Accountability, rapidity of change, complexity, and people mistakes are factors that make controlling an important function in today's organizations. These four controlling factors are briefly explained.

Setting standards, comparing performance to standards and taking corrective action are three stages in the control process. Each of these stages is discussed and a good definition of standards is given.

Health and fitness managers need to be concerned about seven instruments of control available to them, since each of these instruments has a profound effect on the program. However, the budget is one of the most powerful.

Budgets have three important functions. For health and fitness managers, the two direct concerns of budgets are (1) how to obtain the necessary resources to realize the goals of the program and (2) how to use the process of budget development and management to utilize most effectively those resources that are made available to the program.

Three types of budgets are described: line item, performance and program. Line budgeting may be combined with performance or program budgets. Five approaches to developing budgets and determining allocations to organizational units or program components point out the importance of understanding both the techniques and politics involved.

Health and fitness managers should come to the realization that developing a budget and determining allocations, when appropriate, need to be considered carefully.

The two most commonly tried "rational" approaches to budgeting have been planning, programming and budgeting, a centralized approach to budget decision making and zero budgeting, which is more decentralized in character. Health and fitness managers should certainly become aware of program(s) costs, particularly long-term costs.

Once allocation decisions are made, an approved budget is then established for the health and fitness program: Naturally, the manager is responsible for budget management over the course of the fiscal year. Managerial accounting involves collecting financial transaction data through a management information system and generating reports which enable managers to control performance and auditing.

Six bromides for success for good budget development and management are listed and briefly discussed. These may help health and fitness managers obtain and make the best use of available resources.

Evaluation is critical to health and fitness programs: evaluation of the program, the staff and the participants. Program evaluation are both formative and summative. Both of these types are essential in the evaluation of the program(s). Participants enrolled in health education programs are evaluated by pre-testing and post-testing. Some health education tests are standardized, while others are instructor prepared. In both types of tests, the instructor is seeking either general or specific information. Participants enrolled in fitness programs are evaluated on their present fitness level and the progress made toward reaching a satisfactory level upon completion of a program(s). They, too, may wish to be post-tested. Fitness evaluation includes testing of specific areas so that goals may be attained.

Finally, various types of analysis of physical measurements taken from a fitness evaluation are discussed. Also, two examples of the use of data collected may help managers better to understand how to use fitness data.

Chapter XII

THE FUTURE OF HEALTH AND FITNESS PROGRAMS

INTRODUCTION

What is the future of health and fitness programs? This question has been asked many times by top management, executive directors, managers and staff members. Should forecasting the future of health and fitness programs be based on hunches, intuition or guesswork? The answer to this question is, *absolutely not.*

Does the American public understand what good health practices and fitness activities are all about? Do federal, state and local efforts to educate the average citizen about health and fitness seem to be paying off? Are people beginning to take care of themselves in a more intelligent manner and are they able to make quality decisions about spending their money for better health? Is top management convinced that employees who participate in health and fitness programs are less likely to be absent from work, more likely to stay with the job, more likely to perform their work better, more likely to have improved morale and less likely to have medical problems?

This chapter will attempt to answer some of these questions. However, it should be noted that because health and fitness programs are in their infancy and more research needs to be conducted, some of these questions may not be answered until sometime in the future.

GROWTH OF HEALTH AND FITNESS PROGRAMS

Never in the history of America has there been more publicity on health and fitness. "Television, radio, books, newspapers, and magazines are filled with advice, discussions, and warnings about health."[94] The

---

94. Arthur J. Barsky, M.D., *Worried Sick: Our Troubled Quest for Wellness* (Boston, MA: Little, Brown, 1988), p. 87.

heightened awareness of people in the United States concerning their health and physical well-being is causing health and fitness programs to grow, and undoubtedly they will continue to grow. Although the growth of these types of programs has not been explosive, a moderate rate of growth is, perhaps, better.

At this point in the discussion, it seems appropriate to present documented evidence from various sources that health and fitness programs in the United States are growing:

> Approximately five million people went to a health spa last year, up 400,000 from five years ago, and projections are 30 million guests annually in five to ten years.[95]

> Johnson and Johnson estimates some 10,000 organizations offer some form of health promotion programs to business, ranging from insurance companies to local YMCAs to community hospitals.[96]

> Health clubs. Some 7 million Americans, most between the ages of 25 and 44, last year spent $5 billion membership fees to swim, grunt on exercise equipment and play racquetball.[97]

> Institutional sales of fitness equipment should increase by 7 percent annually for the rest of the decade, says FIND/SVP, a research firm, with the fastest growth in sales to corporations and hospitals.[98]

> ...85 million Americans participate in exercise programs.[99]

Although this section concerns growth of health and fitness programs, growth is quite evident in other ways and areas:

> Various market researchers estimate that Americans spend more than $10 billion a year on diet drugs, exercise tapes, diet books, diet meals, weight-loss classes, fat farms and devices like body wraps. Roughly $800 million alone goes for frozen diet dinners and entrees. More than $400 million is rung up for services and products carrying the Weight Watchers name. . . . [100]

> After President Eisenhower suffered coronary damage, this incident: . . . started the nation toward a day when it would include 102 million swimmers, 72 million bicyclists, 34 million runners, 25 million tennis players, 19 million skiers and enough splashy health clubs and old-

---

95. Anastasia Toufexis, "Shake a Leg, Mrs. Plushbottom," *Time*, 127: 78, June 2, 1986.

96. Patricia Winters, "J and J Sees Future in Health Programs," *Advertising Age*, 58:17, 38, April 20, 1987.

97. David Brand, "A Nation of Healthy Worrywarts?" *Time*, 132:4, 66, July 25, 1988.

98. Bryant Robey, "Life On A Treadmill," *American Demographics*, 7:6, 4, June, 1985.

99. Ibid., p. 4.

100. N.R. Kleinfield, "The Ever-Fatter Business of Selling Thinness," *The New York Times*, 135:46890, 1, September 7, 1986.

fashioned gyms to keep 35 million devotees of physical conditioning equipment in workout clothes.[101]

Sears, Roebuck, which advertised a primitive rowing machine in its 1920s mail-order catalog, has devoted 31 pages of its all-winter catalogs to home-fitness devices.[102]

Brand adds the following information:

Equipment. Americans last year bought $138 million worth of exercise benches, light weights, exercise bikes and treadmills for their homes. A decade earlier sales were only $5 million.

Athletic shoes. In 1987 Americans spent $6 billion on brand names, such as Reebok and Nike—three times what they spent in 1977.

Diet food. About $74 billion worth of low-calorie foods, from crackers to nondairy creamers, will be bought in the U.S. this year. That is a third of the nation's total food-store bill.

Vitamins. Manufacturers sold vitamins and minerals worth $2.1 billion in 1987. Sales of calcium and iron supplements are growing faster than those of multivitamins.[103]

Cobb adds:

Doctor Kenneth Cooper's book, *Aerobics,* and its four sequels in print in the United States have sold over 7.5 million copies and the book has been reprinted in 33 languages.[104]

HEALTH OBJECTIVES FOR THE YEAR 2000

It seems appropriate in this chapter to provide health and fitness managers and their staffs with a draft of the priority areas of the national health objectives for the year 2000.

Priority Areas:

1. Reduce Tobacco Use
2. Reduce Alcohol and Other Drug Abuse
3. Improve Nutrition
4. Increase Physical Activity and Fitness
5. Improve Mental Health and Prevent Mental Illness
6. Reduce Environmental Health Hazards
7. Improve Occupational Safety and Health
8. Prevent and Control Unintentional Injuries
9. Reduce Violent and Abusive Behavior

101. Nathan Cobb, "A Nation Getting Into Shape," *Boston Globe,* 23:122, 1, May 1, 1988.

102. Anastasia Toufexis, "Working Out In A Personal Gym," *Time,* 127:6, 74, February 10, 1986.

103. Brand. *Healthy Worrywarts,* p. 66.

104. Cobb, *Getting Into Shape,* p. 20.

10. Prevent and Control HIV Infection and AIDS
11. Prevent and Control Sexually Transmitted Diseases
12. Immunize Against and Control Infectious Diseases
13. Improve Maternal and Infant Health
14. Improve Oral Health
15. Reduce Adolescent Pregnancy and Improve Reproductive Health
16. Prevent, Detect, and Control High Blood Cholesterol and High Blood Pressure
17. Prevent, Detect, and Control Cancer
18. Prevent, Detect, and Control Other Chronic Diseases and Disorders
19. Maintain the Health and Quality of Life of Older People
20. Improve Health Education and Access to Preventive Health Services
21. Improve Surveillance and Data Systems[105]

VALUES RELATED TO HEALTH AND FITNESS PROGRAMS

Of what consequence are good health and a satisfactory level of fitness? What are the values related to health and fitness programs? Because we are now living in a society that is health and fitness conscious, managers and their staffs should become familiar with the values related to health and fitness programs. These programs:

- Create a positive attitude toward a healthy life-style
- Encourage participation in the program(s)
- Provide a health-risk appraisal with feedback
- Provide screening for hypertension, cholesterol level, hearing and glaucoma
- Provide educational programs on stress management, nutrition and weight management, smoking cessation and drug and alcohol abuse
- Improve muscle tone, posture and overall energy
- Reduce chronic fatigue
- Conduct classes for certification in cardiopulmonary resuscitation and first aid
- Provide continuing health education programs, and
- Provide continuing fitness programs in aerobics and weight training.

---

105. Office of Disease Prevention and Health Promotion, National Health Information Center (ONHIC), Washington, D.C., April 3, 1989.

HOW TO FORECAST THE FUTURE OF
HEALTH AND FITNESS PROGRAMS

Managers of health and fitness programs will definitely want to know what the future holds for their types of programs. The question arises, How does one forecast the future of health and fitness programs? Perhaps the technique most appropriate is the Delphi Technique.

> The Delphi Technique is a method for the systematic solicitation and collation of judgments on a particular topic through a set of carefully designed sequential questionnaires interspersed with summarized information and feedback of opinions derived from earlier responses.[106]

The key to the Delphi process as used here is that experts in the field of health and fitness respond independently to the survey question, What is the future of health and fitness programs? After the responses are analyzed, the results are distributed back, in an anonymous way, to the experts, with other follow-up questions which may have surfaced. The experts have the opportunity to modify and/or expand on their original responses predicated upon new information summarized from the judgments sent in by other panel members. This process is repeated through several cycles until a final answer to the original question is derived from a panel of experts.

FUTURE TRENDS IN HEALTH AND FITNESS MANAGEMENT

The future of health and fitness management appears to be bright because there are millions of Americans participating in health and fitness programs who want quality programs with trained, knowledgeable managers. The following sections address three areas that are bound to surface in the future:

Unions*

Regardless of the type of organization, the manager will be responsible for a number of personnel-related issues. These will occur whether the employees are represented by a union or the personnel policies have

---

106. Andre L. Delbecq, Andrew H. Van de Ven and David H. Gustafson, *Group Techniques for Program Planning* (Glenview, IL: Scott, Foresman, 1975), p. 10.

*This section was written by George Hackett, formerly Director of Labor Relations, University of Southern Maine, Portland, Maine.

been developed by management. It should also be expected that there may be differences in some policies applicable to different classifications of employees. Some policies by federal, or in some instances by state, law must be equivalent regardless of classification.

If employees are represented by a union, the right to organize and be represented will be based on federal law, the National Labor Relations Act, in private organizations; and on state law for public organizations. Not all states have adopted statutes providing representation in public organizations, but in some states without such statutes, representation has been recognized.

There are probably many arguments about whether there are differences when employees are represented or not, but two can clearly be identified. With management-developed personnel policies, these can generally be changed without notice and without consultation with employees. Such changes, and interpretations of policies, may be subject to challenge in the courts, often a time-consuming and expensive procedure; and such policies have been recognized by the courts as a contract with employees. Some organizations do provide for an employee advocate or ombudsman to represent employees in situations resulting from changes in policies or interpretations of policies. In an organization with represented employees, it should be recognized that many of the interests of employees are now represented by an agent that is external to the organization in which the employee works. This generally limits what the employees can negotiate for themselves, for the union will now represent the employees on many issues, including disputes with management. Such disputes may result in grievances and subsequently arbitration hearings where decisions can be binding on both parties.

Does a manager approach the two situations differently? The answer to this question may be yes and no, but there are more reasons to answer no than yes. First, regardless of the origin of any personnel policies, management interprets the policies. As noted above, though, the interpretations are subject to challenge, either in the courts or through a grievance procedure. Second, regardless of origin, the language of most personnel policies is generally less than precise. This often occurs in collective bargaining as a compromise for the definitive language proposed by the two parties. At the same time, some policies are best developed with less than precise language to permit manager judgment from one situation to another. Generally, manager decisions cannot be arbitrary and capricious.

Where employees are represented, an organization/union contract may be a more comprehensive set of policies than those developed solely by management, and undoubtedly the union would argue that employees have more rights as a result of a negotiated agreement. This may or may not actually be the case, but management decisions are now monitored by an employee-designated agent. This does not suggest the administrator should make decisions with this in mind, but some decisions will be more closely monitored. These will include in particular any disciplinary action taken, the filling of position vacancies, changes in work schedule, the assignment of overtime opportunities, and the safety and health of employees.

Possibly most management and union disagreements arise over the issue of discipline. With represented employees, the manager will generally be expected to have "just cause" for any action and be able to establish that any discipline is warranted with confirmed facts about a situation. Excluding certain recognized offenses as stealing from the employer, using alcohol on the job, and insubordination as "just cause" for termination, the manager will be expected to use some form of progressive discipline with the employee for minor offenses. The traditional use of this principle would include an oral warning, a written reprimand, and suspension for successive offenses; but it must also include some plan to help the employees to change the behavior that results in the discipline. The number of years the employee has been with the organization and past performance must also be considered in any disciplinary action.

Prior to taking any action, an impartial investigation should be conducted to determine in fact that some offense has occurred. This might appropriately be done by another manager in the organization to preclude that an employee's immediate supervisor functions as investigator, prosecutor, and judge in such circumstances.

In filling position vacancies, current employees will almost always be given some right to a priority consideration, and, in some instances, a right to a vacancy. Any discretion is absent where a right to a vacancy exists; but where a priority consideration is required, the manager must consider any internal candidates. The person selected as the best qualified may be from outside the organization. If, however, an internal candidate is selected, this might be subject to challenge by an employee with greater seniority. In this situation the more senior candidate would generally have to establish having better qualifications for the position than those possessed by the individual selected. Where two or more internal applicants are the best qualified and have substantially similar qualifications, contracts will usually require that the most senior employee be selected.

Probably few, if any, aspects of the employment relationship would be more disruptive to an employee than a change in schedule. Management typically retains the right to control employees and make decisions about the operation of the organization. With a union contract the manager can expect that the interests of the employee must be heard; and if the change in schedule would be too much of a hardship, the employee may well be given some rights based on seniority to retain a current schedule. This may not be within the same unit of the organization, a transfer would be necessary, and it may not be at the same job classification level.

Many employees covet the opportunities for overtime. This often adds significantly to salary or wages. Excluding emergency situations where an available and qualified employee must be quickly offered the chance for the overtime, most union contracts will provide for some equitable distribution of these opportunities. This most likely will be some rotation starting with the most senior employee in a department. The definition of emergency situations may be subject to challenge by the union, and management should be able to establish this fact as related to a particular situation.

Air quality, computer display screens, employee smoking, arrangement of furniture and equipment, and many other possible characteristics of the work place can impact on the health and safety of employees. It is management's responsibility under most contracts to assure a healthy and safe work environment. Many federal and state statutes also address this issue. In fact, it is an accepted labor/management principle that an employee can refuse to work in a location or at a task when there is a threat to the employee's health and/or safety. The judgment about whether a threat exists is often subject to interpretation, but the burden of establishing that it does not is management's.

Other areas that may be considered are non-discrimination, past practice, reclassification, performance review, abuse of sick leave, seniority, and sexual harassment. However, space will not allow for these areas to be discussed.

Gender Preference in Fitness Programs

When organizations are planning to start a fitness program(s) or if such programs are already being conducted, managers should have a general idea as to what programs females prefer and what programs males prefer. Accordingly, the National Sporting Goods Association has published a participation study, January–December, 1988, which reveals the female and male fitness activities preference data. The data are presented below in thousands and in age ranges from under twelve to sixty-five plus.

FITNESS ACTIVITIES:	FEMALE UNDER 12	12-17	18-24	25-34	35-44	45-54	55-64	65+
Aerobic Exercising	679	1768	4056	6874	4060	1479	742	900
Calisthenics	478	1258	1555	1831	1320	500	372	710
Exercise Walking	1038	2132	3928	9256	7890	5658	5356	5999
Exercise With Equipment	186	1288	2990	3771	2573	1569	1013	831
Running/Jogging	844	2146	2399	2035	1313	487	236	100
Swimming	4850	5831	5986	8561	6293	2605	2327	2205
MALE								
Aerobic Exercising	166	182	922	994	665	352	176	172
Calisthenics	304	880	1065	1528	798	362	368	299
Exercise Walking	805	1033	1751	3630	3837	3110	3443	3440
Exercise With Equipment	76	2017	3529	3987	2541	1278	754	537
Running/Jogging	702	2047	3167	3573	2254	1095	284	238
Swimming	4789	5523	5244	7032	4749	2478	1349	1283

Source: Used with permission of the National Sporting Goods Association, Mt. Prospect, Illinois.

Common Fitness Injuries*

With increased participation in a variety of fitness programs throughout the country, inevitably there is an increase in the likelihood of musculoskeletal injuries. Most injuries that occur in organized fitness programs tend to be chronic in nature due to the type of exercise programs offered and the amount of supervision that is required. Most chronic injuries can be avoided or limited in severity with the proper

---

*This section was written by Ellen van Haasteren, Fitness Injury Specialist, University of Southern Maine, Portland, Maine.

education of preventative measures and proper initial treatment. It is important that the staff in any fitness program not evaluate or diagnose injuries but rather be aware of potential harmful exercises that predispose a participant to injury. Moreover, from a managerial perspective, becoming familiar with the common fitness injuries may prove helpful, particularly if managers are involved with fitness instruction.

Shoulder Injuries

Shoulder injuries tend to be quite common in swimming and weight-lifting programs. Impingement of the supraspinatus tendon and the tendon against the acromion and ligament is caused during repetitive use of the arm and shoulder over the head, such as in the freestyle and butterfly stroke in swimming, and the lifting of heavy weights over the head, such as with the shoulder-press exercise with weight lifting.

The impingement causes swelling and inflammation in the joint, which causes pain and weakness in the shoulder area. Tenderness is usually felt just beneath the distal end of the clavicle but may also be more generalized throughout the shoulder area and upper arm. Pain is also felt when the arm is raised to the side past the parallel position. Any activity in which resistance is exerted with the arm overhead, such as the top of the butterfly or crawl stroke, will cause pain. Despite the pain that is experienced, most often there is no visual swelling because the affected area is deep in the shoulder joint.

This injury can be prevented if the proper precautions are taken. Proper shoulder warm-up and cool down are critical to the care of the shoulder. One should never use hand paddles for swimming in the pool unless he or she is an elite swimmer. The general population cannot accommodate to the added resistance and still maintain proper mechanical form. If a swimmer is experiencing any pain in the shoulder, he or she should switch to a stroke that does not involve bringing the arms over the head until the pain subsides. Once the pain has subsided, the participant can gradually start using strokes overhead again.

Over-the-head exercises in weight training should be monitored very carefully. If proper weight progression is not followed with these exercises, especially the shoulder press, the muscles are impinged and overstressed resulting in a tendinitis or impingement injury.

Thoracic Outlet Syndrome

Thoracic outlet syndrome is often seen in weight lifters and caused by the narrowing of the space through which an individual's arteries, veins, and nerves enter his arm. Many anomalies may cause this problem, such as cervical ribs, a cervical vertebra, or a clavicular fracture callus; but often a shoulder drooped from heavy use may be the causative factor.[107] Oftentimes, weight lifters have a muscular imbalance in their shoulder muscles, with overdeveloped chest and anterior shoulder muscles and weak upper back and posterior shoulder muscles. This imbalance, poor posture and drooping shoulders cause a narrowing of this space.

Symptoms of a thoracic outlet problem are general arm swelling and stiffness, cool, pale limb, tingling or numbness; the arm also may feel weak and heavy and tire easily.

It is important that the participants with these problems have them checked out by a doctor to rule out other problems such as a cervical disk problem and so forth. Treatment of thoracic outlet syndrome due to muscular imbalances and poor posture are exercises to strengthen the upper back and posterior shoulder and to re-educate the participant on proper postural alignment.

Groin Strain

The groin strain, probably one of the most common injuries, tends to take a long time to heal and to strengthen. Often, participants try to return to fitness participation before the muscle is properly healed. This muscle group is usually strained because of disregard to proper warm-up stretching before the participant attempts a faster speed, high knee lift or a pivoting turn. The symptoms of this type of strain are a sharp pain in the groin area and inability to flex the hip. Relief is felt if pressure is applied to the affected area.

It is extremely important to ice the area initially and to stretch the affected muscle. Once the pain and swelling have subsided, progressive strengthening can be started with knee lifts and straight leg raises. Stationary bike riding is also very effective in strengthening these muscles. The groin should continue to be iced down after exercise to alleviate the chances of tendinitis occurring.

---

107. Daniel N. Kulund, M.D., *The Injured Athlete* (Philadelphia, PA: J.B. Lippincott, 1982), p. 262.

Chondromalacia

Chondromalacia is probably one of the most common fitness injuries to the knee and is associated with the roughening of the back surface of the kneecap. Pain is usually described as an unexplainable pain behind the kneecap which is exaggerated when pressure is applied. If the leg is fully extended and the participant is asked to tighten the thigh, a sharp pain and a grinding sensation are usually experienced behind the kneecap. Any type of deep knee bend or flexion and extension of the knee may cause pain or grinding. Walking up or down stairs or hills can also be painful to the area.

The treatment, depending on the severity, is usually rest for a period of time to reduce the pain. Full leg extension exercises with resistance and biking can aggravate the knee and should be avoided. Often, physical therapy may be prescribed by a physician to strengthen the quadriceps without aggravating the knee joint. Ice after exercise will often help reduce the swelling and, therefore, some of the pain in mild cases of chondromalacia.

IT Band Friction Syndrome

The iliotibial band runs from the lateral part of the hip to the lateral portion of the tibia just below the knee joint. IT band friction syndrome is common during running and cycling, as this band rubs back and forth on the lateral aspect of the knee causing a bursitis formation. The symptoms of this injury are pain on the lateral side of the knee, especially when the knee is flexed to about 30 degrees.[108] The injury is usually caused by an increase in mileage, running on uneven surfaces, running around a track or course in the same direction, downhill running, or biking with toe clips turned inward. It is important to assess the cause of this injury and change the program accordingly.

Shinsplints

Shinsplints is a catchall term for lower leg pain and is usually defined as an inflammation at the insertion of the muscles to the tibia (shinbone). Many new participants in a walk/jog or aerobics program experience this injury because of the unaccustomed stress to the muscles of the lower leg. It is important to have this injury treated initially to avoid the

---

108. Steven Roy, M.D., and Richard Irvin, *Sports Medicine: Prevention, Evaluation, Management, and Rehabilitation* (Englewood Cliffs, NJ: Prentice-Hall, 1983), p. 432.

possibility of stress fractures which would limit exercise for weeks or months.

Anytime a participant complains of shinsplints, it is advisable to have him or her decrease the intensity and duration of the exercise. Alternating between a stationary bike and walking may decrease the recovery time of the injury, yet the participant may still enjoy the benefits of exercise. If decreasing the intensity and duration does not cause decrease in pain, it is advisable to stop walking altogether and consult a physician to assess the cause of the shinsplints. There may be a biomechanical abnormality that may be causing the problem.

Stress Fractures

Stress fractures can develop in a variety of different areas, such as the feet, lower legs, and hips. These fractures are defined as slight cracks in the bone surface caused by overuse. A sign of a stress fracture is pain associated with palpation to the bone, with no history of trauma. There may be some swelling in the surrounding areas, but there is usually little or no pain with non-weight-bearing exercises. A stress fracture to the hip area is rare but can occur in a program such as walk/jog when a participant has significantly shorter legs than his or her walking partner. The person with the shorter legs tends to overstride, causing added stress to the hip joint. This type of injury is not as common with mismatched walkers as with mismatched runners. Participants should be made aware, though, of the potential of injury when overstriding. Often, a stress fracture in the hip area has the same symptoms as a groin strain, but no history of trauma. There may also be radiating pain down the front of the leg and knee. Besides the pain of stress fractures being very limiting in an exercise program, if gone untreated, a stress fracture can eventually become a complete fracture with very serious complications.

Plantar Fasciitis

Plantar fasciitis is a tear to the ligament in the arch of the foot at the insertion into the heel. The pain is felt under the heel bone, and the first step out of bed in the morning is usually extremely painful. This injury can be caused by trauma, such as a sudden turn or twisting of the foot, or it can have a more gradual onset and be caused by poor arch support, stiff-soled shoes, or a biomechanical abnormality.

Pain upon palpation to the bottom of the foot can cause extreme pain. It is very important to treat this injury early. If not treated properly, it may form a calcium deposit (heel spur), causing a much longer recovery time or even surgery.

Spinal Conditions

Any complaints of spinal column pain should be referred to a physician for evaluation because of the complexity of this region. Before a potential participant starts an exercise program, if he or she experienced some back pain, a note from the physician should explain which exercises to avoid.

FUTURE TECHNOLOGY

Computers in Health and Fitness*

Health and fitness activities have taken the nation by storm. Computers, likewise, are the tools of the life-styles of the nineties and beyond. Both are indicative of Americans' attempting to maintain healthy, active lives while providing for more leisure time in which to do so. Physical activity enables the average American to enjoy a healthier life than previously enjoyed, while the computer complements enjoyment by freeing up time to participate in these activities.

While health and fitness programs are complemented by the computer and vice versa in the modern life-style, use of the computer as a tool to monitor and modernize the management of health and fitness programs is still barely perceptible in most such programs. We are not talking about the *Rocky IV* movie type usage where the Russian boxer is depicted as a computer-developed automation; rather, we are talking about management and monitoring activities that would streamline the day-to-day management of health and fitness programs. In more specific terms, we are talking about using the computer to establish data bases for health risk evaluation results, interest and needs survey results, individual participant health and fitness profiles, financial management and budgets, program information, statistical analysis, and graphics associated with health and fitness programs.

---

*This section was written by Lawrence Braziel, Director, Management Information Systems, University of Southern Maine, Portland, Maine.

Word Processing

The fastest and most useful way to begin using a computer is with the word processing software that can be run on microcomputers. Such software allows the program manager not only to write and edit letters and other communications with relative ease but, also, with the mail-merge and text-merge aspects of most modern word processing software, to make multiple copies of the same letter with personalized salutations and envelopes. Thus, a manager can develop a data file of names and addresses of those enrolled in his or her program, write a letter about a schedule change in the program, and merge the letter with the names file to produce individualized letters to each enrollee, along with individualized envelopes. This not only personalizes the health and fitness program but also becomes a powerful marketing tool for future programs.

We do not recommend one word processor over another (each must be weighed against what the manager wishes to achieve), though we personally like a package for the IBM PC and its compatibles called "Volkswriter 3" by Lifetree Software. This package is relatively simple to learn and use and has quick on-screen help menus available if one gets hung up on what to do next. The Apple MacIntosh world, of course, has its own word processors, any of which might serve well; but the "MacWrite" from Apple Software is as good as any for general usage.

Data Base Management

Data base management software is probably the next most important use of computers. With the proper software, one can register, bill, monitor, and report on all aspects of health and fitness programs. These programs run from the relatively simple "card file" to the more complex "relational" data bases. The card file programs are outstanding for maintaining lists of participants or suppliers. They can be seen to work basically like the "Rolodex" card filing system. "Cardex," a shareware program (low cost commercial software filed in the public domain as a marketing method), is a good example of such a program. The relational data bases are probably the more familiar commercial products similar to Ashton-Tate Corp.'s dBASE III software, or the shareware program "PC File+" by ButtonWare, Inc. Again, with data base management programs, the health and fitness program manager can maintain information on his or her clientele for reporting, accounting, and measuring progress in the programs.

Spreadsheets

Most of us have heard of Lotus Corp.'s "Lotus 123" or other spreadsheet packages. These are data bases set up with matrix format which allow for entering and retrieving information similar to an accounting journal. This spreadsheet format is the basis for commercial accounting and bookkeeping software. The business functions of any office are well served by this type of software, and it is most commonly used for maintaining accounts. However, in health and fitness programs, this format might also be useful for modeling health improvement or maintenance programs, as the spreadsheet is a very powerful projection tool, especially in answering "What if?" questions.

Other Software

The health and fitness program manager may need to use other types of software, depending upon his or her program. There is a wide variety of packages available from communications software, which enable connection with data bases or computers at other sites, through several statistical measurement packages, which let the more statistically oriented manager produce chi-squares and functional-analysis clusters to his or her heart's content.

Public Domain/Shareware Software

While there is much good commercial software available, usually it comes with a fairly stiff price tag. Many health and fitness programs do not have the luxury of purchasing the $300–$1000 software package. Fortunately, there is something called public domain and shareware software. Public domain is software produced by programmers for the sheer challenge of doing so. Most PD's believe that software is for everyone and that there should be no charge for a program. These types of programs are many times very technically strong but weak in documentation and support. A number do have problems which the user is left to his or her own devices to solve.

Shareware is commercial software which usually cannot afford to compete or find marketing outlets through the normal commercial channels. Shareware is put into the public domain for user review. One can use and copy the software to determine if it meets a particular need. If a shareware package does meet a need, then the user will be expected to send in the enclosed license request form and a relatively inexpensive licensing fee to purchase the software. In return, the software's developer will send back a license to use the software (required by federal law) and a reference manual and will provide a support hotline to help solve problems.

Both public domain and shareware software may be obtained for a nominal fee (usually $5–$10 a diskette) to let a computer user review available software applications. A couple of places to contact (but by no means the only places) for copies of shareware diskettes are Public Brand Software, P.O. Box 51315, Indianapolis, Indiana, 46251, for shareware and The Boston Computer Society, Inc., One Center Plaza, Boston, Massachusetts, 02108 (the latter is especially good for various types of computer-related information and services). Other very good sources of computer software information are the local computer clubs. Members are usually more than willing to share knowledge of their experiences with software programs. In many cases, technical support is also available.

Equipment

So far we have been discussing software use. But what about the computer itself? Isn't it the most important part of computing? The answer is, of course, yes and no. The computer is only as good as the software which runs on it, but the software is only as good as the computer it can run on. Now that we are confused, let me explain.

Computers come in all sizes and varieties. When shopping at your local computer store, such phrases as 286 chips, 386 chips, laser printers, mouse, EGA, VGA, etc. will fly heavily around the room. These will be interspersed with single-user, multi-user, networked, partitioned disks, and the like. Quickly, it becomes obvious that the uninitiated user will be overwhelmed with the technical jargon and not know what to do. This will be followed by intense stress and long delays as the health and fitness manager studies and restudies his or her budgets, thinks through various options, and dreads making the decision which may or may not be the wrong choice. Well, these stresses and anxieties can be relieved by putting together a strategy for looking at equipment and approaching the purchasing process.

First, before going to look at equipment, develop a plan or list of what things you need a computer for. This will take a little review of the software available (*PC Magazine, PC World, MacWorld, Byte* are a few of the computer-oriented magazines available at most bookstores) and discussions with some computer users to decide what such equipment may be used for. This will take some effort on the manager's part, but the results will be a better understanding of how computers may be used in health and fitness. Also, talk to peers and colleagues who have already invested time in moving into computing, getting both success and horror stories in order to know what to expect. Next, decide who and how many people are going to use the computer(s) system you need. Will it just be a single user system (one person entering and retrieving information from the computer) or multiple users (the entire staff, maybe)? Finally, and most importantly, take a computer friend or even hire a business-oriented computer club member or consultant to go with you to translate what all these terms mean; however, try to make sure this friend or consultant is not going to be encouraging you to get the latest or most cutting edge of what is on the market. You don't need to be the vanguard; you need to make the system work for your program. By going well prepared, you will be assured of not only cutting through much of the technical jargon but also of getting the best and the most computer necessary to manage your program.

Computers and their accompanying software applications are invaluable tools to all managers. Health and fitness program managers will receive the same benefits as any other manager. Using computers with appropriate software will more efficiently maintain the business functions of the programs, while more specific software will enable the monitoring of participants' progress in the programs. Any manager of a health and fitness program should take advantage of the computer as a tool to enable better delivery and quality of his or her programs in order to complement better his or her roles as the provider for healthy lifestyles for the present and the future.

New Trends in Fitness Equipment*

When health and fitness managers take a look at any advertisement or manufacturer's information for contemporary exercise equipment, one thing becomes very clear: the use of computers (and their accompanying technologies) is, and will be, moving into all aspects of exercise equipment and routines. Video monitors, digital displays, and voice synthesizers coupled with computers especially designed for efficient exercise regimens provide the participant with an individualized picture of the effectiveness of his or her exercise program. Exercise equipment is now

---

*This section was also written by Lawrence Braziel.

available which uses computer microchip technology not only to monitor the progress of the participant but also to provide competitive challenges to make the exercise routine an intriguing test between the participant and the computerized opponent. This not only makes today's equipment and exercise more fun but also encourages a more regular use of the equipment. Thus, exercise equipment is moving away from the "20 minutes on the bike is good for everyone" philosophy toward a program designed and monitored specifically for each individual participant.

Principal pieces of equipment that presently use some form of computerized monitoring include exercise stairs, treadmills, stationary bicycles, all types of weight training hardware, and rowing machines. Riding a stationary bike is no longer the boring task it used to be. With computer technology and video monitors, the bike becomes part of a biking road race game, as it takes one along a peaceful mountain road with trees and valleys stretching ahead, while the rider has never left the comfort of the fitness club. Additionally, the rider receives constant updating on speed, distance, calories burned, and other motivational information to assist him or her in meeting certain goals.

Computerized treadmills and stairs are available with digital displays that also show time, speed, calories burned, and resistance, as well as provide pace information. All information and exercise parameters are electronically adjusted to meet the individual's exercise goals. These aerobic conditioners have control panels by which one inputs and controls resistance and incline of the treads.

Some computerized rowing equipment comes with sound effects and computer-produced graphics which show two racing scull boats, one belonging to the participant, the other to the computer competitor. The intensity of this race can be adjusted to meet the physical conditioning and goals of the participant. This system, which is used to build cardio-respiratory endurance, involves interval training techniques, such as the racing graphics and pacesetting techniques. Other features include calories burned per hour, timing indicators, difficulty and duration monitors, and stroke counting.

Strength training equipment is available which uses computer microchip technology to emulate weight training resistance and can be personalized for a participant's exercise program. These chips are "burned" (permanently programmed) with instruction sets that tell the computer in the weight training equipment to provide a specified amount of resistance. Instead of adding 5- and 10-pound weights, the participant keys in on the control panel the amount of weight desired and the equipment provides the proper resistance. The programs can also do pre-training measurements of strength to help tailor each participant's workout routine. Additionally, range of motion is established, and resistance patterns are monitored to work specific muscle groups. As with the other pieces of exercise equipment, certain actions, such as repetitions and time, are recorded.

In the not too distant future, this microchip concept will most likely be extended to IC cards (microchip memory cards not unlike those used in some automatic teller machines or in security lock systems) which can be individualized, with each person's exercise regimen programmed into the card at relatively moderate cost. The participant will be able to carry such a card in his or her wallet and use it anywhere there is a compatible exercise machine. Thus, personalized exercise regimens, whether at the club or at the gymnasium, will become easier and more beneficial as programs are formulated for the individual, meeting his or her own special requirements. This will assure the traveling businessperson or anyone else away from the "home" club or gymnasium that wherever he or she is, the individually designed exercise routine will be available.

The more common use of exercise computers has been to emulate mechanical equipment while keeping track of such measurements as elapsed time, caloric use, distance and the like. The coming trend for this equipment will be to monitor digitally heart rates, blood pressure, body temperature, muscle fatigue, and other fitness indicators to develop a totally tailored health and fitness program using the new exercise equipment. Fitness goals will be input into the exercise computer, and the equipment will maintain the levels of exercise recommended. For example, a participant might have a fitness regimen established that involves use of a computerized treadmill. The parameters of effort which the individual should achieve, but not exceed, are stored in the computer. The computer then monitors vital signs, such as heart rate, blood pressure, and body temperature, to minimize the possibility of the person's overdoing. The treadmill, in turn, adjusts speed and resistance to maintain the level of effort as recommended in the participant's exercise program; it can even shut down if the user fails to heed the warnings of the monitoring system. With today's computer technology and advances, the monitoring system may employ either digital displays (video screens and monitors) or voice simulation (the machine speaks to the participant) with the use of appropriate computer chips and speakers. Just as some automobiles tell you, "Your door is open," the exercise equipment of the near future will ask you to "Please slow down. You are exceeding your recommended heart rate."

The new high technology exercise equipment is taking the world of fitness and exercise by storm. Computer chips, video screens, digital displays, and voice and audio simulators provide monitoring and motivation for the exercise regimen. Barely touching the surface of possibilities, the exercise equipment of the future will surely become increasingly sophisticated. Personalized programs will be developed that will monitor the total fitness needs of the individual; and the exercise equipment, with its computerized control, will be programmed to provide a whole plan designed for the individual participant. Surely, the future world of fitness will be exciting, with more improvements to come.

SUMMARY

Health and fitness programs in America have been growing at a moderate rate. There has been much publicity about such programs by various media and there will be more to come.

The National Health Objectives are listed. These objectives will provide managers with the priority areas for the year 2000 and may serve as a base for future programming.

In most cases participants will want to know what values are related to health and fitness programs. The values were listed so that managers and their staffs may reacquaint themselves with them.

All health and fitness managers, whether they are novice or experienced, will want to know what the future has in store for their programs. The Delphi Technique is a tool that will help them forecast this future.

Managers can expect that unions, gender preference in fitness programs, and common fitness injuries are areas that will need a considerable amount of their attention. These areas are bound to surface in the future and, as a consequence, will require trained and knowledgeable staff and managerial personnel.

The chapter culminates with a discussion on computers in health and fitness and new trends in fitness equipment. Managers should become familiar with both these topics, as computers and newly designed fitness equipment will be in the limelight in the years ahead.

APPENDICES

Appendix A
(Sample)

EMPLOYEE HEALTH INTEREST SURVEY*

This survey is optional and strictly CONFIDENTIAL, for health promotion program planning purposes only.

A. EXERCISE

1. What is your major form of regular exercise? (CIRCLE ONE)
   - (a) None (skip to question 4)
   - (b) Bicycling
   - (c) Team sports
   - (d) Aerobics/aerobic dance
   - (e) Brisk walking
   - (f) Jogging/running
   - (g) Racquetball/tennis
   - (h) Swimming
2. How many times a week do you usually exercise?
   - (a) Once or less
   - (b) Twice
   - (c) 3–4 times
   - (d) 5 times or more
3. How long do you exercise at a time?
   - (a) Less than 15 minutes
   - (b) 15–20 minutes
   - (c) 20 or more minutes
4. If you are not exercising regularly now, please circle why:
   - (a) Too inconvenient
   - (b) Don't like physical exercise
   - (c) Not enough time
5. If exercise programs were organized for employees, which type of program would you be interested in joining? (CIRCLE ONE)
   - (a) Not interested
   - (b) Running/jogging
   - (c) Walking
   - (d) Bicycling
   - (e) Aerobics/aerobic dance
   - (f) Swimming
   - (g) Team sports
   - (h) Tennis/racquetball
6. If intramural sports were organized for employees, which type of program would you be interested in joining? (CIRCLE ONE)
   - (a) Not interested
   - (b) Volleyball
   - (c) Softball
   - (d) Basketball
   - (e) Golf
   - (f) Bowling
   - (g) Soccer
   - (h) Racquetball/tennis
   - (i) Track and field

---

*Note: Reproduced with permission by Center For Health Promotion, Osteopathic Hospital of Maine, Inc., Portland, Maine.

7. How do you prefer to exercise? (CIRCLE ONE)
   - (a) On my own
   - (b) Informally with friends
   - (c) Formal group

8. If exercise programs were offered, please indicate the most appropriate time you would attend: (CIRCLE ONE)
   - (a) Not interested
   - (b) Before work
   - (c) During lunch
   - (d) Immediately after work
   - (e) Evenings
   - (f) Saturday
   - (g) Sundays

B. WEIGHT MANAGEMENT/NUTRITION

1. Do you consider yourself to be overweight?
   - (a) Yes
   - (b) No

2. How many pounds overweight do you consider yourself to be?
   - (a) Less than 10 lbs.
   - (b) 10–20 lbs.
   - (c) More than 20 lbs.

3. Which of the following weight management programs are you participating in at the present time? (CIRCLE ONE)
   - (a) None
   - (b) Weight Watchers
   - (c) Diet Workshop
   - (d) Nutri-System
   - (e) Overeaters Anonymous
   - (f) My own diet plan
   - (g) Private nutritionist
   - (h) Exercise

4. If a formal weight management program was organized for employees would you participate?
   - (a) Yes
   - (b) No

5. If a weight management program was offered, please indicate the most appropriate time you would attend: (CIRCLE ONE)
   - (a) Not interested
   - (b) Before work
   - (c) During lunch
   - (d) Immediately after work
   - (e) Evenings
   - (f) Saturdays
   - (g) Sundays

6. Do you eat breakfast?
   - (a) Yes
   - (b) No

7. Do you eat three or more meals per day?
   - (a) Yes
   - (b) No

8. Do you eat a balanced diet? (Eating foods from the Basic Four food groups—Fruit and Vegetables, Dairy Products, Carbohydrates, Protein)
   - (a) Yes
   - (b) No

9. Are you aware that experts recommend limiting the amount of salt, sugar, and fat in the diet?
   - (a) Yes
   - (b) No

C. SMOKING CESSATION

1. Do you smoke?
   (a) Yes   (c) No, I quit
   (b) No

2. Do you support the organization's smoking policy?
   (a) Yes   (c) Not sure
   (b) No

3. If you are a smoker, would you be interested in participating in a quit-smoking program if more were offered to employees? (CIRCLE ONE)
   (a) No   (d) Yes, I prefer a group
   (b) Yes, I prefer an individual   program
       program   (e) Yes, I prefer a video tape
   (c) Yes, I prefer a self-help   program
       (booklet) program

4. If a group smoking cessation program was offered, please indicate the most appropriate time you would attend: (CIRCLE ONE)
   (a) Not interested   (e) Evenings
   (b) Before work   (f) Saturdays
   (c) During lunch   (g) Sundays
   (d) Immediately after work

D. STRESS MANAGEMENT

1. How often do you feel that you are under a lot of stress?
   (a) None of the time   (d) Most of the time
   (b) Rarely   (e) All of the time
   (c) Sometimes

2. How often do you feel tense?
   (a) None of the time   (d) Most of the time
   (b) Rarely   (e) All of the time
   (c) Sometimes

3. What do you feel contributes to your stress most of the time? (CIRCLE UP TO THREE AREAS)
   (a) Family   (f) Lack of fitness
   (b) Work   (g) My own coping style
   (c) Finances   (self-concept)
   (d) Poor eating habits   (h) Social pressure
   (e) Interpersonal relationships

4. What do you do to manage stress? (CIRCLE ALL THAT APPLY)
   (a) Nothing   (d) Talk to friends, relations
   (b) Exercise   (e) Time management
   (c) Relaxation techniques

5. If a group stress management program was offered, please indicate the most appropriate time you would attend: (CIRCLE ONE)
   (a) Not interested   (e) Evenings
   (b) Before work   (f) Saturdays

(c) During lunch   (g) Sundays

(d) Immediately after work

6. Would you be interested in participating in a stress management program?

   (a) No

   (b) Yes, I prefer an all-day group program

   (c) Yes, I prefer four two-hour sessions with follow-up

   (d) Yes, I prefer a self-help program

   (e) Yes, I prefer a videotape program

7. At work what causes the greatest stress? (CIRCLE ONE)

   (a) Stress at work is not significant

   (b) Lack of training

   (c) Physical environment (light, noise, temperature, etc.)

   (d) Unrealistic deadlines

   (e) Relation to employees (supervisor/subordinates/peers)

   (f) Communication (inaccurate, muddled feedback)

   (g) Limited advancement

   (h) Lack of recognition for good work

E. BLOOD PRESSURE

1. Have you had your blood pressure taken in the last year?

   (a) Yes   (b) No

2. Have you ever been told by a doctor that you have high blood pressure?

   (a) Yes   (b) No

If YES, please answer 3, 3a, and 4; If NO, please go on to questions about OCCUPATIONAL HEALTH & SAFETY.

3. Are you currently being treated by a doctor for high blood pressure?

   (a) Yes   (b) No

3a. If yes, by what method(s) of treatment? (CIRCLE ANY)

   (a) Medication   (d) Weight reduction

   (b) Exercise   (e) Changes in eating habits

   (c) Stress management

4. Is your blood pressure now within normal limits?

   (a) Yes   (b) No

F. OCCUPATIONAL HEALTH & SAFETY

1. Do you have concerns about the following issues/problems in your work environment?

   (a) Yes   (b) No   (1) Noise

   (a) Yes   (b) No   (2) Chemicals

   (a) Yes   (b) No   (3) Overcrowding

   (a) Yes   (b) No   (4) Hot and cold environment

   (a) Yes   (b) No   (5) Lifting heavy objects

   (a) Yes   (b) No   (6) Eyestrain

   (a) Yes   (b) No   (7) Indoor air quality

(a) Yes   (b) No   (8) Equipment related hazards (excluding vehicles)

(a) Yes   (b) No   (9) Automobile hazards

2. Can you identify a person or persons responsible for occupational health and safety for your work environment?

   (a) Yes   (b) No

3. Do you see the need for an occupational health and safety person or committee to address health and safety hazards in your work environment?

   (a) Yes   (b) No   (c) Do not know

G. HEALTH INFORMATION SERIES

If a lecture and discussion series were organized for employees, which of the following topic areas would you participate in?

1. Nutrition
   - (a) Sugarless eating, sugar substitutes
   - (b) Dieting sensibly, safely
   - (c) Meatless meals
   - (d) Cooking for one or two
   - (e) Nutritional fast food (cooking on the run)
   - (f) Low cholesterol, low salt, low fat cooking
   - (g) Prenatal nutrition
   - (h) Caffeine and your health
   - (i) Food additives, reading labels

2. Stress Management
   - (a) Dealing with emotions (depression, anger)
   - (b) Making decisions
   - (c) Assertiveness training/communication
   - (d) Dealing with loneliness
   - (e) Relaxation techniques
   - (f) Time management
   - (g) Career development
   - (h) Balancing work and home

3. Self-Care (Taking Care of Yourself/Family)
   - (a) Treating the common cold
   - (b) Dental health
   - (c) When to seek medical attention
   - (d) When to seek counseling
   - (e) Accident prevention
   - (f) Prevention of childhood illnesses
   - (g) Choosing a physician
   - (h) How to choose day care

4. Physical fitness
   - (a) Healthy back program
   - (b) Yoga
   - (c) Choosing an exercise program (all your favorites)
   - (d) Beginning and maintaining an exercise program
   - (e) Exercising safely
   - (f) Office exercise
   - (g) Prenatal/postnal exercise
   - (h) Nutrition and the athlete

5. Adult Health Issues
   - (a) Reproductive health/birth control
   - (g) Parenting
   - (h) Mid-life crisis

(b) Rape and Rape Prevention

(c) Cancer

(d) Sexually transmitted diseases

(e) Breast self-examination

(f) Managing menopause

6. Occupational/Environmental Issues
   (a) Chemical exposure (dioxin, EDB's, etc.)
   (b) Safety tips with household chemicals, poison prevention
   (c) Video display terminals
   (d) Gardening organically
   (e) Work place design

7. Alcohol and Other Drugs
   (a) Know your medications
   (b) Drug education for parents (not for parents only)
   (c) Developing healthy alternatives to alcohol/drug abuse
   (d) Drinking and driving
   (e) Alcohol, drugs, and pregnancy
   (f) How to talk to any kid about drugs

(i) Predictable life stages

(j) Self-esteem

(k) Dealing with loss (i.e., divorce/death)

(l) Caring for an elderly parent

(f) Nuclear power/radiation

(g) Identifying occupational/environmental health hazards

(h) Noise pollution

(i) Radon in water

(g) Help for the alcohol/drug abusers and those affected

(h) Myths about alcohol and other drugs

(i) Children of alcoholics

(j) How to be a positive influence on a smoker's quit effort

8. If health information workshops were offered, please indicate the most appropriate time you would attend: (CIRCLE ONE)
   (a) Not interested
   (b) Before work
   (c) During lunch
   (d) Immediately after work
   (e) Evenings
   (f) Saturdays
   (g) Sundays

H. GENERAL INFORMATION
(CIRCLE ONE ANSWER PER QUESTION)

REMINDER: This survey and your answers are optional and strictly CONFIDENTIAL. The answers are to be used for program planning purposes only.

1. How old are you?
   (a) 18–24 years
   (b) 25–34 years
   (c) 35–44 years
   (d) 45–54 years
   (e) 55–64 years
   (f) 65+ years

2. Are you?
   (a) Male
   (b) Female

3. Are you?

(a) Married no children
(b) Married with dependent children

(c) Single
(d) Single parent

4. Where is your work location?

(a) ————————————————
(b) ————————————————

5. Which shift do you work?

(a) Day
(b) Evenings

(c) Nights
(d) Rotating shifts

6. Can you take your lunch/dinner break at different times?

(a) Yes

(b) No

7. How much time do you usually take for lunch/dinner?

(a) 30 minutes or less
(b) 45 minutes

(c) 60 minutes
(d) 60+ minutes

8. What time do you normally start your lunch/dinner break?

(a) 11:00 a.m.
(b) 11:30 a.m.
(c) 12:00 noon
(d) 12:30 p.m.
(e) 1:00 p.m.

(f) 1:30 p.m.
(g) 5:30 p.m.
(h) 6:00 p.m.
(i) 6:30 p.m.
(j) 7:00 p.m.

9. If you have dependents living with you, what age are they?

(a) Infant
(b) Toddler
(c) Preschool
(d) Elementary

(e) Adolescent
(f) Adult
(g) Elderly

Appendix B*

PARTICIPANT NEEDS ASSESSMENT FORM

(This is a sample questionnaire. You will probably have to modify this form to obtain the exact information you would like to analyze.)

A. Check the items you would like to improve.
_____ Your Health
_____ Your Fitness Level
_____ Your Weight/Appearance
_____ Your Energy Level

B. Are you currently involved in any regular activity or program designed to improve or maintain your health?
Yes _____   No _____

C. If yes, check the activities in which you participate and the times of day they occur.
_____ Walking
_____ Jogging
_____ Cycling
_____ Exercise classes
_____ Aerobic dance
_____ Weight training
_____ Racquetball
_____ Tennis
_____ Health education seminars
_____ Other activities (please list)

_____

_____

Times: Before work   _____
        Mid-morning   _____
        Lunchtime   _____
        Mid-afternoon   _____
        After work   _____

D. If offered, would you participate in a company-sponsored health/fitness program on a regular basis?
very likely _____   likely _____   not likely _____

*Note: Reproduced with permission from the Exercise Program Coordinator's Guide, American Heart Association.

E. If activities could be offered by the company, which would interest you the most and what times during the day would you participate?

_____ Walking
_____ Jogging
_____ Cycling
_____ Exercise classes
_____ Aerobic dance
_____ Weight training
_____ Racquetball
_____ Tennis
_____ Health education seminars
_____ Other activities (please list)

_____

_____

Times: Before work   _____
         Mid-morning   _____
         Lunchtime   _____
         Mid-afternoon   _____
         After work   _____

F. If other aspects of the program could be offered, which would interest you the most and what times during the day would you participate?

_____ Blood pressure screening
_____ Smoking cessation
_____ Nutrition education
_____ Weight control classes
_____ Other activities (please list)

_____

_____

Times: Before work   _____
         Mid-morning   _____
         Lunchtime   _____
         Mid-afternoon   _____
         After work   _____

G. Would you be willing to share the cost of health/fitness programs?
   very likely _____   likely _____   not likely _____

H. If likely, to what financial extent?

   $1 per week   _____ $5 per class   _____
   $5 per week   _____ $10 per class   _____
   $50 per month _____ $20 per class   _____

I. To what extent should your spouse be involved in the health/fitness program?
   High _____   Medium _____   Low _____   Not at all _____

J. To what extent should your children be involved in the health/fitness program?
   High _____ Medium _____ Low _____ Not at all _____

K. Would you participate in medical screening tests if offered?
   very likely _____ likely _____ not likely _____

L. Would you be willing to share the cost of the medical screening tests?
   very likely _____ likely _____ not likely _____

M. If likely, to what financial extent?

   $5 per test _____ $10 per test _____
   $20 per test _____ $50 per test _____
   $100 per test _____ $200 per test _____

N. What other suggestions do you have concerning a health/fitness program?

   _____
   _____
   _____

JOB DESCRIPTION

I. *Title:*
II. *Organizational Relationships:*
   A. *Reports to:*
   B. *Supervises:*
   C. *Coordinates with:*
III. *Primary Purpose of Position:*
   A. *Major Duties of Position:*
   B. *Secondary Duties:*
IV. *Budget Responsibilities:*
V. *Public and Professional Activities Related to Job Performance:*
VI. *Knowledge and Skill Qualifications:*
   • *Required:*
   • *Preferred:*
   • *Desired:*
VII. *Job Classification:*
   Level _____
   Salary Range:

*Courtesy of the University of Southern Maine, Portland, Maine.

LINE BUDGET

Item	*Current Budget*	*Actual*	*Proposed*
Salaries and Wages			
Fringe Benefits			
Supplies and Materials			
Rent			
Utilities			
Equipment			
Postage			
Travel			
Depreciation			
Data Processing			
Printing			
Maintenance			
Miscellaneous			

Appendix E
(Sample)

PERFORMANCE BUDGET

Item	*Current Budget*	*Actual*	*Proposed*
Fitness Testing			
General			
Physical Rehabilitation			
Cardiac Rehabilitation			
In-Service Training			
Manager(s)			
Program Coordinator(s)			
Fitness Staff			
Health Education Staff			
Fitness Testing Technician(s)			
Secretary(ies)			
Services			
General Fitness Class(es)			
Physical Rehabilitation Class(es)			
Cardiac Rehabilitation Class(es)			
Health Education Class(es)			

PROGRAM BUDGET

Item	Current Budget	Actual	Proposed
Health Education			
Environmental Management			
Nutrition and Weight Management			
Smoking Cessation			
Stress Management			
Substance Abuse: Alcohol and Drugs			
Fitness			
Aerobic Dance			
Aerobic Exercise			
Aquatic Fitness			
Walk/Jog			
Weight Training			
Timed Calisthenics			
Flexibility			
Cardiac Rehabilitation			
Pulmonary Rehabilitation			
Low Back Rehabilitation			

Appendix G*
(Sample)

STAFF EVALUATION FORM

NAME: _____

DATE: _____

POSITION: _____

I. PERSONAL QUALITIES. (Rate each quality below by selecting the phrase most closely describing the staff member's actual performance.)

---

1. *Appearance.* (Consider appearance during contact hours.)

___	___	___	___	___	___
Not Observed	Unsatis-factory	Below Average	Satis-factory	Very Good	Out-standing

---

2. *Initiative.* (How well does he/she begin an assignment and then carry it through without direction?)

___	___	___	___	___	___
Not Observed	Must usually be told exactly what to do	Relies on others; needs help getting started	Does regular work without prompting	Proceeds on assigned work voluntarily & readily accepts suggestions	Self-starter; makes practical suggestions

---

3. *Attitude.* (Observable attitudes toward job environment.)

___	___	___	___		___
Not Observed	Unsatis-factory	Below Average	Satis-factory	Enthusiastic	Outstand-ing; very positive

---

*Note: Reproduced with permission by University of Southern Maine's Health and Fitness Program— Lifeline.

4. *Leadership.* (Consider ability to accomplish objectives by directing and/or working with peers, subordinates, participants.)

___	___	___	___	___	___
Not Observed	Fails to command; unable to exert control	Manages in some instances to obtain effective cooperation	Develops adequate cooperation & teamwork under normal circumstances	Commands respect of associates; effective even under difficult circumstances	Has outstanding skills in giving directions; inspires confidence even under very difficult circumstances

5. *Cooperation.* (How well does he/she get along with others?)

___	___	___	___	___	___	___
Not Observed	Refuses to cooperate or to give help	Sometimes creates friction; slow to help others	Most relations with others are harmonious under normal circumstances	Pleasant to work with even in difficult situations	Always works in harmony with others; an excellent team worker	Extremely successful in working with others; actively promotes harmony

6. *Attendance.* (Consider all absences and tardiness unexcused and excused.)

___	___	___	___	___	___
Not Observed	Frequent absences; often late	Occasionally absent or late, usually with good reason	Satisfactory	Very Good	Outstanding

7. *Judgment.* (Consider consequences of decisions made.)

___	___	___	___	___	___
Not Observed	Decisions or recommendations are wrong more	Prone to neglect or misinterprets facts; com-	Judgment usually sound &	Judgment consistently results from sound eval-	Outstanding sound and logical thinker

often than right	mits occa- sional errors in judgment	reasonable	uation of all the factors involved	with an exceptional grasp of the situation involved

II. PERFORMANCE QUALITIES.

1. *How much is known about assigned duties?* (Consider the technical "know-how," knows what to do; knows the required steps.)

Not Ob- served	Lacks knowledge of simplest duties	Knows only the very routine duties	Knows all routine duties with some knowledge of more com- plex duties	Has ex- tensive knowledge of complex duties	Has mas- tered all duties.	Has master- all duties & has extensive knowledge of related positions

2. *How well are assigned duties accomplished?* (Consider the following: a careful worker; a thorough worker; checks work.)

Not Ob- served	Fails more often than suc- ceeds	Slow & sometimes inatten- tive, but completes routine duties with fair results	Completes most as- signed duties satis- factorily	Completes all assigned du- ties satis- factorily	Consist- ently produces very high quantity & quality work	Succeeds where others would fail; quality & quantity of work consis- tently out- standing

3. *Quality of work.* (How accurate, neat, complete is the work?)

Not Observed	Inaccurate & careless	Occasionally careless; needs check- ing	Work is acceptable	Careful worker; seldom needs correction	Consistently neat, accurate & thorough

4. *Quality of work.* (How much satisfactory work is turned out by the staff member?)

Not Observed	Inadequate turnout of work	Inclined to be slow	Does suffi- cient amount of work	Usually does more than expected	Maintains unusually high output

5. *Safety.* (How well does the staff member demonstrate a concern for safety, i.e. emergency procedures?)

Not ob-served	Shows little concern for safety	Occasionally careless; needs further guidance	Works in a safe manner avoiding acci-dents & in-juries	Has con-cern for safety of self, other employees, & members.	Strives to improve and & make positive recommend-ations re-lative to improvement of unsafe conditions

6. *Housekeeping.* (Consider appearance of work area.)

Not Observed	Unsatis-factory	Below Average	Satisfactory	Very Good	Outstand-ing

7. *Communication Facility.* (Consider ability to accomplish objectives through oral and written communication.)

Not Observed	Unable to express thoughts clearly; lacks or-ganization	Expresses thoughts satisfact-orily on routine matters	Organizes and expresses thoughts clearly & concisely on routine mat-ters	Excellent command of writ-ten & oral ex-pression; consist-ently able to express ideas clearly	Outstanding ability to communicate ideas to others through written & oral ex-pression

8. *Relationship to participants* (How well does this staff member relate to participants?)

Indifferent and unresponsive	Responsive if asked or directed	Relates well to all parti-cipants	Usually makes a special effort to relate to	Outgoing, sensitive, & ade-quately res-

	participants			ponsive to participants under all circumstances	

9. *What effort is made for self-improvement?* (Consider efforts to improve educational level or technical knowledge appropriate to program needs.)

_____	_____	_____	_____	_____	_____
_____	_____	_____	_____	_____	_____
Not Observed	Rejects opportunities	Shows little desire to take advantage of opportunities	Usually accepts opportunities given	Frequently seeks out opportunities to improve self	Outstanding motivation & energy in seeking out & using opportunities

III. GENERAL QUALITIES.

1. *How well does he/she utilize resources?* (Consider ability to utilize effectively money and materials.)

_____	_____	_____	_____	_____	_____	_____
_____	_____	_____	_____	_____	_____	_____
Not Observed	Ineffective in the conservation of materials & economical use of manpower	Utilizes money & materials in a barely satisfactory manner	Usually conserves money & materials by implementing & maintaining routine management procedures	Almost always effective in accomplishing savings in money & materials by improving management procedures	Always effective in accomplishing savings in money & materials by developing improved management procedures	Exceptionally effective in the utilization of money and materials

2. *How well is responsibility accepted?* (Consider whether responsibility is taken for own actions, the actions of subordinates and the objectives of the program(s).)

_____	_____	_____	_____	_____	_____	_____
_____	_____	_____	_____	_____	_____	_____
Not Observed	Fails to accept	Accepts some re-	Accepts most responsi-	Accepts all as-	Takes initi-	Assumes full res-

major responsibilities specifically assigned	sponsibilities when specifically assigned	bilities when specifically assigned	signed responsibilities	ative to to assume added responsibilities when necessary to meet an objective	ponsibility for meeting objectives even when not specifically assigned

IV. FUTURE EVALUATION DATES.

Date of next evaluation _____.

Date of special interim evaluation (if indicated) _____.

_____   _____
Manager   Date

I have read and understand the contents of this evaluation.

_____   _____
Staff Member   Date

BIBLIOGRAPHY

Allen, Louis A. "Managerial Planning: Back to Basics." *Management Review*, 70:4, 15–20, April, 1981.

Allen, Robert F. "The Corporate Health-Buying Spree: Boon or Boondoggle?" *Advanced Management Journal*, 45:2, 5–22, Spring, 1980.

"A.M.A. Board Approves New Marketing Definition." *Marketing News*, 19:3, 1, March, 1985.

American College of Sports Medicine, *Guidelines For Exercise Testing and Prescription*, 3rd ed. Philadelphia, PA: Lea & Febiger, 1986.

Arnold, John D. "The Why, When, and How of Changing Organizational Structures." *Management Review*, 70:3, 17–20, March, 1981.

Baird, John E. Jr. "Supervisory and Managerial Training through Communication by Objectives." *Personnel Administrator*, 26:7, 28–32, July, 1981.

Barker, Ben D., John M. Lowe, and Robert D. Sparks. *Viewpoint: Toward A Healthier America*. A summary report on health issues and related programming activities of the W. K. Kellogg Foundation, Battle Creek, MI: January, 1980.

Barnes, Lan. "AAFDBI: Bringing Fitness to Corporate America." *The Physician and Sports Medicine*, 11:2, 127–133, January, 1983.

Barsky, Arthur J., M.D. *Worried Sick: Our Troubled Quest for Wellness*. Boston, MA: Little, Brown, 1988.

Baun, William B. and Michele Baun. "A Corporate Health and Fitness Program. Motivation and Management by Computers." *Journal of Physical Education, Recreation and Dance*, 55:4, 42–45, April, 1984.

Bechtel, Stefan. "Wellness in the Work Place." *Prevention*, October, 1982.

Bedeian, Arthur G. and William F. Glueck. *Management*, 3rd ed. New York, NY: The Dryden Press, 1983.

Bedworth, Albert E. and David A. Bedworth. *Health For Human Effectiveness*. Englewood Cliffs, NJ: Prentice-Hall, 1982.

Bensinger, Peter B. "Drugs in the Workplace." *Harvard Business Review* (Special Report), 60:6, 48–60, November–December, 1982.

Berkowitz, Eric N., Roger A. Kerin and William Rudelius. *Marketing*. St. Louis, MO: Times Mirror/Mosby, 1986.

Bernotavicz, Freda and Miriam Clasby. *Competency Across the Campus: The University Secretary*. Portland, University of Southern Maine, 1984.

Blackburn, Richard S. "Dimensions of Structure: A Review and Reappraisal." *The Academy of Management Review*, 7:1, 59–66, 1982.

Blake, Robert R., and Jane S. Mouton. *The Managerial Grid*, III, 3rd ed. Houston, TX: Gulf, 1985.

Boone, Louis E., and David L. Kurtz. *Principles of Management*, 2nd ed. New York, NY: Random House, 1984.

Bradford, David L., and Allan R. Cohen. *Managing For Excellence: The Guide To Developing High Performance in Contemporary Organizations.* New York, NY: Wiley, 1984.

Brand, David. "A Nation of Healthy Worrywarts." *Time*, 132:4, 66–67, July 25, 1988.

Brennan, Andrew J.J. "A Corporate Health Advocate Shares His Fiscal Findings." *Personnel Administrator*, 27:4, 39–42, April, 1983.

Brennan, Andrew J.J. "Health Promotion in Business: Caveats for Success." *Journal of Occupational Medicine*, 23:9, 639–642, September, 1981.

Brennan, Andrew J.J. "How To Set Up A Corporate Wellness Program." *Management Review*, 72:5, 41–47, May, 1983.

Brennan, Andrew J.J. (Guest Editor). "Worksite Health Promotion." *Health Education Quarterly.* New York, NY: Human Sciences, 1982, 9:, Special Supplement, Fall, 1982.

Briggs, Tom. "Industry Starts To Take Fitness Into The Plant." *Executive*, 5:25, February, 1975.

Briscoe, Dennis R. "Organizational Design; Dealing with the Human Constraint." *California Management Review*, 23:1, 71–80, Fall, 1980.

Bucher, Charles A. *Administration of Physical Education and Athletic Programs*, 8th ed. St. Louis, MO: Mosby, 1983.

Bureau of Health, Maine Department of Human Services, and Blue Cross and Blue Shield of Maine. *Guidelines For Choosing Worksite Health Promotion Programs.* November, 1984.

Carroll, Charles, and Dean Miller. *Health: The Science of Human Adaptation*, 3rd ed. Dubuque, IA: Brown, 1982.

Chen, Moon S., Jr. "Wellness in the Workplace: A Review of the Literature." *Health Values: Achieving High Level Wellness*, 6:5, 14–18, September/October, 1982.

Cheney, Paul H., and Gary W. Dickson. "Organizational Characteristics and Information Systems: An Exploratory Investigation." *Academy of Management Journal*, 25:1, 170–184, 1982.

Cherrington, David J. *Organizational Behavior.* Boston, MA: Allyn and Bacon, 1989.

Christopher, William F. "Is the Annual Planning Cycle Really Necessary?" *Management Review*, 70:8, 38–42, August, 1981.

Clutterbuck, D. "Executive Fitness Aids Corporate Health." *International Management*, 35: 19–22, February, 1980.

Cobb, Nathan. "A Nation Getting Into Shape." *Boston Globe*, 233:122, 1, 20, May 1, 1988.

Cohen, William S. "Health Promotion in the Workplace." *American Psychologist*, 40:2, 213–216, February, 1985.

Collings, Jr., G.H. "Health, A Corporate Dilemma; Health Care Management, A Corporate Solution," In *Springer Series on Industry and Health Care.* New York, Springer-Verlag, 3: 16–28, 1977.

Cook, Ronald J., Richard T. Walden and Donald D. Johnson. "Employee Health and Fitness Program at the Sentry Corporation." *Health Education*, 10:4, 4–6, July/August, 1979.

Daniel, D.W. "What Influences a Decision? Some Results from a Highly Controlled Defense Game." *Omega*, 8: 409–419, November, 1980.

Data Management, "Pressure-Prone Information Managers Can Avoid," 21:9, 24–27, September, 1983.

Davis, Mary F. "Worksite Health Promotion: An Overview of Programs and Practices." *Personnel Administrator*, 29: 45–50, December, 1984.

Dedmon, R.E. et al. "An Industry Health Management Program." *Physician and Sportsmedicine*, 7:11, 57–61, 64–67, November, 1979.

Delbecq, Andre L., Andrew H. VandeVen and David H. Gustafson. *Group Techniques for Program Planning*. Glenview, IL: Scott Foresman, 1975.

Dessler, Gary. *Management Fundamentals: Modern Principles & Practices*, 4th ed. Englewood Cliffs, NJ: Prentice-Hall, 1985.

Dickerson, O.B., and C. Mandelblit. "A New Model for Employer-Provided Health Education Programs." *Journal of Occupational Medicine*, 25:6, 471–474, June, 1983.

Donaldson, Les. *Behavioral Supervision*. Reading, MA: Addison-Wesley, 1980.

Donnelly, Jr., James H., James L. Gibson and John M. Ivancevich. *Fundamentals of Management*, 6th ed. Homewood IL: Irwin, 1984.

Dossett, Dennis L., Carl I. Greenberg. "Goal Setting and Performance Evaluation: An Attributional Analysis." *Academy of Management Journal*, 24:4, 767–779, 1981.

Driver, Russell W., and Ronald A. Ratliff. "Employers' Perceptions of Benefits Accrued From Physical Fitness Programs." *Personnel Administrator*, 27:8, 21–26, August, 1982.

Dunn, S. Watson, and Arnold M. Barban. *Advertising, It's Role in Modern Marketing*, 6th ed. New York, NY: Dryden, 1986.

Edlin, Gordon, and Eric Golanty. *Health & Wellness: A Holistic Approach*. Boston, MA: Science Books, 1982.

"Employee Fitness Shapes Up As A Business," *Business Week* (Industrial Edition), 2695:34B, July 6, 1981.

Fallek, Max. *How To Set Up Your Own Small Business*, 1. Minneapolis, MN: American Institute of Small Business, 1987.

Fallon, William K. (Ed.). *AMA Management Handbook*, 2nd ed. New York, NY: American Management Associations, 1983.

Famularo, Joseph J. (Ed.). *Handbook of Human Resources Administration*, 2nd ed. New York, NY: McGraw-Hill, 1986.

Feldman, Daniel C., and Hugh J. Arnold. *Managing Individual and Group Behavior in Organizations*. New York, NY: McGraw-Hill, 1983.

Fielding, Jonathan E. "Effectiveness of Employee Health Improvement Programs." *Journal of Occupational Medicine*, 24:11, 907–916, November, 1982.

Flamion, Allen, "The Dollars and Sense of Motivation." *Personnel Journal*, 59:1, 51–53, January, 1980.

Flynn, Richard B. (Editor and Contributing Author). *Planning Facilities for Athletics Physical Education and Recreation*. North Palm Beach, FL: The Athletic Institute and Reston, VA: American Alliance for Health, Physical Education, Recreation, and Dance, Revised, 1985.

Fuller, Stephen H. "How To Become the Organization of the Future." *Management Review*, 69:2, 50–53, February, 1980.

Galbraith, Jay R. "Designing the Innovating Organization." *Organizational Dynamics*, 10:3, 5–25, Winter, 1982.

Goldbeck, Willis B. *A Business Perspective on Industry and Health Care.* Springer Series on Industry and Health Care, 2. New York, NY: Springer-Verlag, 1978.

Golding, Lawrence A., Clayton R. Myers and Wayne E. Sinning. *The Y's Way to Physical Fitness; A Guide Book For Instructors.* Revised. Chicago, IL: National Board of YMCA, 1982.

Goldsmith, Seth B. *Health Care Management: A Contemporary Perspective.* Rockville, MD: Aspen, 1981.

Green, Charles N., Everett E. Adam, Jr., and Ronald J. Ebert. *Management.* Englewood Cliffs, NJ: Prentice-Hall, 1985.

Grimaldi, Joseph, and Bette P. Schnapper. "Managing Employee Stress: Reducing the Costs, Increasing the Benefits." *Management Review*, 70:8, 23–37, August, 1981.

Guralnik, David B., Editor in Chief. *Webster's New World Dictionary*, 2nd College Edition. New York, NY: Prentice-Hall, 1986.

Hackman, J.R., G. Oldham, and K. Purdy. "A New Strategy for Job Enrichment." *California Management Review*, 17:4, Summer, 1975.

Haimann, Theo, William G. Scott and Patrick E. Connor. *Management*, 4th ed. Boston, MA: Houghton Mifflin, 1982.

Halcomb, Ruth. "Fitness By Design." *Corporate Fitness & Recreation*, 3:4, 18–20, 23, 25, and 27, June/July, 1984.

Halcomb, Ruth. "Survival of the Fittest: How to Succeed in Corporate Fitness and Recreation." *Corporate Fitness & Recreation*, 3:5, 6, 35–39, August/September, 1984.

Hax, Arnoldo C., and Nicolas S. Majlug. *Strategic Management: An Integrative Perspective.* Englewood Cliffs, NJ: Prentice-Hall, 1984.

Hersey, Paul, and Ken Blanchard. *Management of Organizational Behavior: Utilizing Human Resources*, 4th ed. Englewood Cliffs, NJ: Prentice-Hall, 1982.

Howard, Ann, and Douglas W. Bray. "Today's Young Managers: They Can Do It, But Will They?" *The Warton Magazine*, 5:4, 23–28, Summer, 1981.

Hubsch, Donald M. "Planning the Staffing of a Growing Business." *Management Review*, 70: 59–61, August, 1981.

Hunsaker, Phillip L., and Johanna S. Hunsaker. "Decision Styles—In Theory, In Practice." *Organizational Dynamics*, 10:2, 23–36, Autumn, 1981.

Ivancevich, John M., James H. Donnelly, Jr. and James L. Gibson. *Management for Performance: An Introduction to the Process of Managing.* Homewood, IL: Irwin, 1983.

Iwan, Eula. "How to Conduct an Interest Survey," Employee Services Management, Westchester, IL: *National Employee Services and Recreation Association*, 28:2, 16–19, March, 1985.

Kahalas, Harvey. "Planning Types and Approaches: A Necessary Function." *Managerial Planning*, 28:6, 22–27, May/June, 1980.

Katz, Robert L. "Skills of an Effective Administrator." *Harvard Business Review*, 52:5, 50–102, September/October, 1974.

King, John L. "Cost-benefit Analysis for Decision-Making." *Journal of Systems Management*, 31: 24–29, May, 1980.

Kleinfield, N.R. "The Ever-Fatter Business of Selling Thinness." *New York Times*, 135:46890, 1, 28, September 7, 1986.

Kondrasuk, Jack N. "Corporate Physical Fitness Programs: The Role of the Personnel Department." *Personnel Administrator*, 29: 75–80, December, 1984.

Kondrasuk, Jack N. "Studies in MBO Effectiveness." *The Academy of Management Review*, 6:3, 419–430, 1981.

Kotler, Philip. *Marketing For Nonprofit Organizations*, 2nd ed. Englewood Cliffs, NJ: Prentice-Hall, 1982.

Kurtz, Norman R., Bradley Googins and William C. Howard. "Measuring the Success of Occupational Alcoholism Programs." *Journal of Studies on Alcohol*, 45:1, 33–45, 1984.

Kuzela, Lad. "Taking a Scalpel to Health-Care Costs." *Industry Week*, 218: 44–46, 50–51, 22, August, 1983.

LaPlace, John. *Health*, 4th ed. Englewood Cliffs, NJ: Prentice-Hall, 1984.

Levine, Edward. "Let's Talk: Breaking Down Barriers to Effective Communication." *Supervisory Management*, 25:6, 2–12, June, 1980.

Levine, Edward L. "Let's Talk: Communicating with the New Worker." *Supervisory Management*, 25:8, 12–23, August, 1980.

Litterer, Joseph A. *Organizations: Structure and Behavior*, 3rd ed. New York, NY: Wiley, 1980.

Littlejohn, Robert F. "Team Management: A How-To Approach to Improved Productivity, High Moral, and Longer Lasting Job Satisfaction." *Management Review*, 71:1, 23–28, January, 1982.

Longe, Mary E., and Donald B. Ardell. "Wellness Programs Attract New Markets For Hospitals." *Hospitals*, 55:22, 115–116 and 119, November, 1981.

Longenecker, Justin G., and Charles D. Pringle. *Management*, 5th ed. Columbus, OH: Merrill, 1981.

Longest, Jr., Beaufort B. *Management Practices for the Health Professional*, 3rd ed. Englewood Cliffs, NJ: Prentice-Hall, 1984.

Lovelock, Christopher H., and Charles B. Weinberg. *Marketing For Public and Nonprofit Managers*. New York, NY: Wiley, 1984.

Lukus, Edmund J. "Strategic Budgeting: How To Turn Financial Records into a Strategic Asset." *Management Review*, 70:3, 57–61, March, 1981.

Lyman, David, Fred Luthans and Nancy Carter. "For Managers in New Jobs: An Accountability and Appraisal System." *Management Review*, 69:1, 46–51, January, 1980.

Malasanos, L., Violet Barkauskas, Muriel Moss and Kathryn Stoltenberg-Allen. *Health Assessment*, 2nd ed. St. Louis, MO: Mosby, 1981.

March, James G. "Footnotes to Organizational Change." *Administrative Science Quarterly*, 26:4, 563–577, 1981.

Maslow, Abraham H. *Motivation and Personality*, 2nd ed. New York, NY: Harper and Row, 1970.

Matteson, Michael T., and John M. Ivancevich. "The How, What and Why of Stress Management Training." *Personnel Journal*, 61:10, 768–774, October, 1982.

McConkey, Dale D. *How to Manage by Results*, 4th ed. New York, NY: American Management Associations, 1983.

Megginson, Leon C., Donald C. Mosely and Paul H. Pietri, Jr. *Management, Concepts and Applications*, 2nd ed. New York, NY: Harper & Row, 1986.

Mescon, Michael H., Michael Albert and Franklin Khedouri. *Management*, 2nd ed. New York, NY: Harper & Row, 1985.

Meyer, Paul J. "Executive Fitness: Time for Exercising." *Sales and Marketing Management*, 126:7, 67–69, May 18, 1981.

Miner, John B., Timothy M. Singleton and Vincent P. Luchsinger. *The Practice of Management*. Columbus, OH: Merrill, 1985.

Mobily, Kenneth. "Using Physical Activity and Recreation to Cope With Stress and Anxiety: A Review." *American Corrective Therapy Journal*, 36:3, 77–81, May/June, 1982.

Mondy, R. Wayne, Robert E. Holmes and Edwin B. Flippo. *Management: Concepts and Practices*, 2nd ed. Boston, MA: Allyn & Bacon, 1983.

Moravec, Milan. "Performance Appraisal: A Human Resource Management System with Productivity Payoffs." *Management Review*, 70:6, 51–54, June, 1981.

Murnighan, J. Keith. "Group Decision-Making: What Strategies Should You Use?" *Management Review*, 70:2, 55–62, February, 1981.

Murr, Donald W., Harry B. Bracey, Jr., & William K. Hill. "How To Improve Your Organization's Management Controls." *Management Review*, 69:10, 56–63, October, 1980.

Nieman, David C. *The Sports Medicine Fitness Course*. Palo Alto, CA: Bull, 1986.

Occupational Outlook Handbook. Washington, DC: U.S. Department of Labor, Bureau of Labor Statistics, 1986.

O'Donnell, Michael P., and Thomas H. Ainsworth. *Health Promotion in the Workplace*. New York, NY: Wiley, 1984.

Oran, Daniel, and Jay M. Shafritz. *The MBA's Dictionary*. Reston, VA: Reston, 1983.

Ostro, Harry. "How Do You Motivate Your Staff?" *Scholastic Coach*, 51:3, 4, 6, 8, 10, and 44, October, 1981.

Owens, James. "A Reappraisal of Leadership Theory and Training." *Personnel Administrator*, 26:11, 75–84, November, 1981.

Parkinson, Rebecca S., and Associates. *Managing Health Promotion in the Workplace, Guidelines for Implementation and Evaluation*. Palo Alto, CA: Mayfield, 1983.

Pearson, Clarence E. "Implementing a Health Promotion Program." *Personnel Journal*, 62:2, 150–154, February, 1983.

Philip, Dorothy M. "Health and Fitness Marketing: Consumers Take Care of Themselves." *Marketing Communications*, 8:11, 30–35, November, 1983.

Pinney, William E., and Donald B. McWilliams. *Management Science, An Introduction to Quantitative Analysis for Management.* New York, NY: Harper & Row, 1982.

Piscopo, John. *Fitness and the Aging.* New York, NY: Macmillan, 1985.

Portland's Parcourse Fitness Circuit. Blue Cross and Blue Shield of Maine, Portland, ME, n.d.

Preventive and Rehabilitative Exercise Committee of the American College of Sports Medicine. *Guidelines for Exercise Testing and Prescription,* 3rd ed. Philadelphia, PA: Lea and Febiger, 1986.

Public Health Service, U.S. Department of Health and Human Services, Office of Disease Prevention and Health Promotion. *The 1990 Health Objectives for the Nation: A Midcourse Review.* Washington, D.C., 1986.

Pyle, Richard L. "Corporate Fitness Programs How Do They Shape Up?" *Personnel,* 56:1, 58–67, January/February, 1979.

Pyle, Richard L. "Performance Measures for a Corporate Fitness Program." *Training and Development Journal,* 35:7, 32–38, July, 1979.

Rees, W. David. *The Skills of Management.* Beckenham, Kent: Croom Helm, 1984.

Richie, Douglas H., Jr. "Aerobic Floor Surfaces." *Corporate Fitness & Recreation,* 5:, 55–59, August/September, 1986.

Rieder, George A. "The Role of Tomorrow's Manager." *Personnel Administrator,* 20:1, 15–19, January, 1975.

Robbins, Stephen P. *Management: Concepts and Practices.* Englewood Cliffs, NJ: Prentice-Hall, 1984.

Roberts, Harold S. *Roberts Dictionary of Industrial Relations,* 3rd ed. Bureau of National Affairs, Washington, D.C., 1986.

Robey, Bryant. "Life On A Treadmill." *American Demographics,* 7:6, 4, 6, June, 1985.

Rosen, Robert H. "The Picture of Health in the Work Place." *Training and Development Journal,* 38:8, 24–30, August, 1984.

Rubinson, Laura, and Wesley F. Alles. *Health Education: Foundations for the Future.* St. Louis, MO: Times Mirror/Mosby, 1984.

Rutman, Leonard, and George Mowbray. *Understanding Program Evaluation.* Beverly Hills, CA: Sage, 1983.

Schermerhorn, John R., Jr. *Management For Productivity,* 2nd ed. New York, NY: Wiley, 1986.

Shepard, Roy J. "Practical Issues in Employee Fitness Programming." *Physician and Sportsmedicine,* 12:6, 160–166, June, 1984.

Shepard, Roy J. "The Economic Benefit of Health and Fitness Programs." *Fitness in Business,* 2:3, 100–104, December, 1987.

Silver, Gerald A. *Introduction to Management.* St. Paul, MN: West, 1981.

Snyder, Neil, and William K. Glueck. "How Managers Plan—The Analysis of Managers' Activities." *Long Range Planning,* 13:1, 70–76, February, 1980.

Spirn, Steven, J.D. and David W. Benfer (Eds.). *Issues in Health Care Management.* Rockville, MD: Aspen, 1982.

Stokes, Linda K., and John C. Rosala. *How Business Can Improve Health Planning and Regulation.* National Chamber Foundation, Washington, D.C., 1978.

Silagyi, Andrew D., Jr. *Management and Performance*, 2nd ed. Glenview, IL: Scott, Foresman, 1984.

Taylor, Robert B. *Health Promotion: Principles and Clinical Applications.* Norwalk, CT: Appleton-Century-Crofts, 1982.

Terry, George R., and Stephen G. Franklin. *Principles of Management*, 8th ed. Homewood, IL: Irwin, 1982.

This, Leslie E. "Critical Issues Confronting Managers in the '80's." *Training and Development Journal*, 34:1, 14–17, January, 1980.

Tolley, Leslie. "Management in the 1980's—Key Issues and Priorities." *Long Range Planning*, 14:1, 55–59, February, 1981.

Tosi, Henry L., and Stephen J. Carroll. *Management*, 2nd ed. New York, NY: Wiley, 1982.

Toufexis, Anastasia. "Working Out In A Personal Gym." *Time*, 127:6, 74–75, February 10, 1986.

Toufexis, Anastasia. "Shake a Leg, Mrs. Plushbottom." *Time*, 127:, 78–80, June 2, 1986.

Tramel, Mary E., and Helen Reynolds. *Executive Leadership: How To Get It & Make It Work.* Englewood Cliffs, NJ: Prentice-Hall, 1981.

Trewatha, Robert L., and M. Gene Newport. *Management.* Homewood, IL: Irwin, 1982.

Tucker, Harvey J. "Budgeting Strategy: Cross-Sectional Versus Longitudinal Models." *Public Administration Review*, 41:6, 644–649, November/December, 1981.

U.S. News and World Report. "A Conversation with B.F. Skinner—Reward or Punishment: Which Works Better?" *U.S. News & World Report*, 89:18, 79–80, November, 1980.

Van Dam, Andre. "The Future of Management." *Management World*, 7:2, 3–6, January, 1978.

Veney, James E., and Arnold D. Kaluzny. *Evaluation and Decision Making for Health Services Program.* Englewood Cliffs, NJ: Prentice-Hall, 1984.

Walton, Eric J. "The Comparison of Measures of Organization Structure." *The Academy of Management*, 6:1, 155–160, 1981.

Weinshall, Theodore D., and Yael-Anna Raveh. *Managing Growing Organizations: A New Approach.* New York, NY: Wiley, 1983.

"Where to Begin: A Basic Guide to Planning An Employee Fitness Program." *Athletic Purchasing and Facilities*, 4:7, 28, 30–31, July, 1980.

Winters, Patricia. "J and J Sees Future In Health Programs." *Advertising Age*, 58:17, 38, April 20, 1987.

World Health Organization. *The First Ten Years of the World Health Organization.* Geneva: World Health Organization, 1958.

Wright, C. Craig. "Cost Containment Through Health Promotion Programs." *Journal of Occupational Medicine*, 24:12, 965–968, December, 1982.

Zieger, Robert H. *American Workers, American Unions, 1920-1985.* Baltimore, MD: Johns Hopkins University Press, 1986.

INDEX